# Body Image Problems
## & Body Dysmorphic Disorder

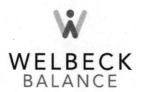

WELBECK
BALANCE

# ABOUT THE AUTHORS

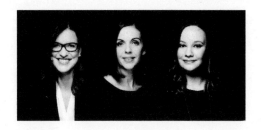

**Lauren Callaghan (CPsychol, PGDipClinPsych, PgCert, MA (hons), LLB (hons), BA)**, is an industry-leading psychologist, and an expert in the field of obsessive compulsive disorders, including BDD. She appeared as a treating clinician in the critically acclaimed and BAFTA award winning documentary *Bedlam*, and is a frequent speaker on radio and TV. Lauren also co-founded the global charity The Shaw Mind Foundation.

**Annemarie O'Connor (CPsychol, DClinPsy, PgCert, BSc)** is a national specialist in treating people with body image concerns and BDD, and OCD. She is a regular speaker at international conferences for BDD, and her opinion is regularly sought for articles, radio pieces and TV programmes about body image issues. Annemarie has also worked with cosmetic surgeons to help them offer appropriate support to people with BDD.

**Chloe Catchpole** has suffered from BDD since her mid-teens. Using the techniques in this book, she has learnt how to manage it and is following her dream of being a writer and film reviewer. Chloe is extremely passionate about raising awareness for Body Dysmorphic Disorder, a little-known disorder which can be utterly debilitating.

# Body Image Problems
## & Body Dysmorphic Disorder
### The Definitive Treatment
### and Recovery Approach

By Lauren Callaghan (CPsychol, PGDipClinPsych, PgCert,
MA (hons), LLB (hons), BA), Annemarie O'Connor (CPsychol,
DClinPsy, PgCert, BSc) & Chloe Catchpole

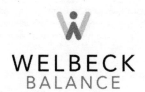

WELBECK
BALANCE

A Trigger Book
Published by Welbeck Balance
An imprint of Welbeck Publishing Group
20 Mortimer Street
London W1T 3JW

First published by Trigger Publishing in 2016

Reprinted by Welbeck Balance in 2021

A CIP catalogue record for this book is available from the British Library

ISBN

978-1-78956-035-0

Cover design by More Visual

Typeset by Fusion Graphic Design Ltd

Printed in Great Britain by CPI Group (UK) Ltd, Croydon CRO 4YY

10 9 8 7 6 5 4 3 2 1

**Note/Disclaimer**

**www.welbeckpublishing.com**

# CONTENTS

# INTRODUCTION

***Chloe:*** When you're 18, the world is your oyster. There are possibilities everywhere you look. It's the start of a whole new life of adventure. Or at least it should be. But it wasn't like that for me. At 18, I was a recluse. While people my age were travelling, starting jobs, or embarking on their first term at university, I was hidden away in one room in my parents' house. I lived in that room. I ate there and I cried myself to sleep there.

If you'd met me, you wouldn't have known why I was so unhappy. You wouldn't have seen what I saw when I looked in the mirror. And you probably wouldn't have heard of Body Dysmorphic Disorder (BDD) – a type of body image problem. I hadn't. Not yet. All I knew was that I wasn't fit to be seen by anyone. When I saw myself, I recoiled at my ugliness. Other people looked at me with absolute disgust – or at least that was what I thought. So I started to hide myself away from the world. I didn't want anyone to see me. I didn't want them to have to suffer because of my ugliness.

My world was growing smaller and smaller. I dropped out of college and took a job at a fast food restaurant, but only managed three weeks there. My parents kept trying to encourage me to get a volunteering job – something to boost my self-esteem and give me a sense of purpose. But it was no good. Aged 18, with my whole life in front of me, I was barely functioning.

I slept a lot. It was the only way to hide the pain. In desperation, Mum arranged for me to have some generic counselling. I talked about the pain in my life and about why I was struggling to cope day-to-day. It was good to talk to someone impartial, but there was no change in my situation. I still believed that I was incredibly ugly and avoided leaving my room whenever I could.

Mum and Dad did everything they could to try to motivate me. They even found a part-time college so I could finish my A Levels, and I tried, I really tried, but it was getting harder and harder to function.

I couldn't talk to anyone. I couldn't explain what was going on in my head, but I knew I had to try. So, in desperation, I wrote Mum a letter:

*I can't really say things face-to-face, so I'll try to say them here. I'll be honest: I really don't want to do my exams. I'm not ready. I think that I need to be in a better place mentally. I should be thinking about how best to revise, but the constant thought on my mind is how I can shut myself away from everyone – and I know that's not right. I'm constantly worried about people looking at me and what they'll think of me. That's why I try to go out as little as possible.*

*Every day is a struggle when you hate the person you see in the mirror. I hated being on the Tube today in London. I saw this girl who was just so beautiful. Everything about her was perfect, and at that moment, I just wanted to be in my bed, hiding away from the world.*

I can still see that girl in my mind's eye. She was everything I wanted to be, whereas I couldn't stand the sight of myself. I was an ugly freak. I knew what people must have thought when they looked at me, because I thought it too. I couldn't stand being seen out in public, so I hid away whenever I was able to.

I felt like I had no future, as if the best years of my life were already long behind me. I was in a dark circle of nothingness; there was no hope, no light. The things I once enjoyed didn't matter any more. Year after year, I would think, *It's going to be different this year*. But it never changed. Over the next few months and the next couple of years, it only got worse.

I was genuinely terrified. I knew I couldn't go on like this. Other people my age were becoming independent and doing whatever they wanted to do. But I felt stuck. I didn't want to die, but I didn't want to live either. I didn't want to *feel* anything. I didn't want to *be* anything. Just being awake was too much for me. It was a constant cycle of feeling ugly, hideous, guilty, and worthless.

I couldn't do anything productive and I didn't feel like I was good at anything. I was a burden on society and a drain on my family. And that's why I slept. I didn't want to think about the reality of my life any more than I had to. I knew that during sleep, I could be free of it all.

When I was younger, I used to wake up with a headful of dreams. But at 18, I didn't remember any dreams when I woke. I just waited for my harsh reality to close in around me again. Sometimes when it was all too much, when I needed to stop all the voices telling me how ugly and useless I was, I would cut myself. Hurting myself physically became my only distraction – it was a way of shutting off my negative thoughts for a few minutes. It was better to focus on the pain than the failure.

I felt like such a let-down – like I was the only one not doing anything with my life. When my dad didn't understand, he'd say, 'You're just being lazy now.' But I was falling lower and lower into a dark pit and I couldn't get out. I couldn't even pretend that I was living a normal life any more. I rarely went outside. I felt like the Hunchback of Notre Dame.

To me, the thought of going out was mortifying. But if I absolutely had to go out, I would look at my feet as I walked, and keep my eyes fixed on the ground. I knew that if I glanced up and saw someone looking at me it'd confirm all my worst fears. I would see them staring at me because they couldn't believe I was so ugly, and it would just be proof that I was right. Mum tried to tell me that people really didn't care what I looked like, that they were just going about their business. But I couldn't believe that. I'd seen all those people looking; I *knew* they were staring, so I just kept on piling up all this evidence, in my head, of how ugly I was.

I knew full well that I was extremely ugly and disfigured. But sometimes – very occasionally – the odd thought would flash through my mind that maybe, just maybe, I was wrong. Maybe my neck didn't stick out, maybe my skin wasn't blemished, and maybe there wasn't hair all over my face. But then I'd see my reflection in a shop window and I'd see that it was actually all true.

That was my life. There was no prospect of getting better. I was destined to live life as a recluse. It was the only way I could be sure I'd keep my hideous features hidden away from other people.

It wasn't until much later, when I was diagnosed with Body Dysmorphic Disorder, that all these things started to make any kind of sense. It was only then that I realised I had a mental illness. It was only then that I had any hope that I might, one day, get better. And then, finally, when I met Lauren and Annemarie and started treatment, things really started to change for the better ...

 **_Lauren:_** As you have heard from Chloe, she had such a miserable existence due to her body dysmorphia that her quality of life was severely compromised. She couldn't do any of the things that most people her age take for granted. Just leaving the house and walking to the local shop was a very distressing ordeal for her. If you suffer with body image problems – what we might also refer to as "body dissatisfaction" – or Body Dysmorphic Disorder (BDD), then I'm sure you will empathise with Chloe's story.

I am so glad you're reading this book. It is a really important and positive first step on your road to overcoming your body image problems, and through this book we will embark on the journey together. I can assure you that you are not alone, and that help and a more positive future are very much within your reach.

In this book, we'll share insights from the work Annemarie and I have done with Chloe, and you may find that you recognise aspects of yourself, or your life, in her story. We'll introduce you to strategies that will help you overcome your body image problems and take back control of your life. Our approach is an effective way of treating body image problems and BDD, and it is accessible to everyone. You don't need any specialist knowledge – this book will give you the tools you need to recover and build a new life for yourself. Our techniques are easy to understand and follow, and deliberately so. We want anyone who is suffering with body image problems or BDD to be able to pick up this book and use it to help them overcome their difficulties.

However, please note, this isn't a quick fix. Your recovery will still take a bit of time and you will need to devote some time and energy to getting better. Don't worry, we're not talking about years and years; we hope that you start to see improvements in weeks! We already know how much effort and energy it takes to live with negative body image issues or BDD, so if you can invest just some of that energy into our approach, you will be able to overcome your body image problems or BDD. Each small, incremental improvement will feel liberating. It will feel like you are getting your life back, bit by bit.

Now, what qualifies me to write this book? Well, to start, I specialise in the treatment of obsessive problems and anxiety disorders, including BDD. I am a clinical psychologist and CBT therapist, trained to deliver psychological treatments that are backed up by scientific evidence – so we know they work! Originally from New Zealand, I now live in London, UK, and I run two practices in London which specialise in a number of conditions including anxiety and obsessional disorders.

Following my clinical psychology training at the University of Canterbury in New Zealand, I moved to the UK and worked at the renowned Centre for Anxiety Disorders and Trauma (CADAT) at the Maudsley Hospital in London. I was part of the National Services Team for OCD and BDD, a UK government-funded programme to treat the most severe cases of OCD and BDD around the country. I am considered a national-level specialist in OCD and BDD, and I teach and supervise psychologists and Cognitive Behavioural Therapy (CBT) therapists, as well as presenting at national and international-level conferences on these topics. I am interviewed regularly for articles, radio pieces and TV programmes about obsessional and anxiety problems and I am a guest lecturer and honorary researcher at the Institute of Psychiatry, King's College.

I am passionate about giving back to the community and promoting evidence-based psychological treatments. I am actively involved in fundraising and supporting OCD and BDD charities in many ways – including raising awareness of obsessional and anxiety disorders – and I present at annual charity conferences for sufferers and their families. Recently I co-founded the Shaw Mind Foundation charity with a former OCD sufferer, Adam Shaw. The Shaw Mind Foundation is focused on reducing the stigma attached to mental health problems, helping those with mental disorders and providing support for their families and friends.

I wanted to write a book on body image problems and BDD to help people suffering from these difficulties, because they often avoid seeking help. They may believe they will be judged as vain, and not taken seriously. BDD is a serious psychiatric condition that requires evidence-based psychological treatment, such as the techniques contained in this book, and may also need medication and specialist input from professionals who specialise in body image issues and BDD. We also live in a world which is increasingly connected and visual. The increase in use of social media and exposure to images in mainstream media heightens a person's awareness of their image and appearance, and this often leads people to compare themselves to "perfect" or "ideal" images. This results in increased body dissatisfaction and body image problems, which, while they might not be diagnosable mental health disorders like BDD, can still significantly affect a person's sense of wellbeing, self-confidence and ability to live their life fully.

It is vitally important that people realise they can take control of how they feel about themselves and their bodies. With this book, you can access the methods that we use when we work with people suffering with body image issues in our practice. With this book, you can learn to accept your appearance and improve your relationship with your body.

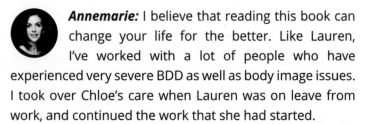

***Annemarie:*** I believe that reading this book can change your life for the better. Like Lauren, I've worked with a lot of people who have experienced very severe BDD as well as body image issues. I took over Chloe's care when Lauren was on leave from work, and continued the work that she had started.

Like Lauren, I am a very experienced psychologist with a number of years' experience working in mental health and assessing and treating a range of psychological difficulties. I met Lauren when we both worked at The Centre for Anxiety Disorders and Trauma (CADAT) team at the Maudsley Hospital. There I also worked in the national specialist treatment team, treating people with BDD and OCD. I have a particular interest in complex anxiety presentations, perfectionism, and communication skills.

Lauren and I decided to join forces and set up a private practice in central London offering specialist services for obsessional and anxiety disorders. We shared a similar way of working, both favoured an evidence-based approach to our work, and wanted to make these methods available for the wider public to access.

I present regularly at international conferences for BDD, attend "ask the expert" forums at support groups for people suffering with body image issues and their loved ones, train cosmetic surgeons in how to help people with BDD and am interviewed regularly for articles, radio pieces and TV programmes about body image issues. All of this is to raise awareness of what can range from unhealthy dissatisfaction with your body to an all-consuming, debilitating illness. Through this book, we hope to continue our campaign to raise awareness.

I know that recovery is possible. It takes effort, of course, but living with BDD takes effort – a lot of effort. And although it may not feel at all possible, change and recovery are within your reach. And we're going to show you how.

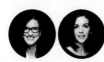 ***Lauren and Annemarie:*** In Part I of this book, you will read Chloe's story. We worked with Chloe to help her

understand her BDD, including how it developed, what kept it going, and how her co-morbid depression impacted on her BDD. We taught her to identify and challenge her unhelpful thinking patterns, accept and tolerate her emotional distress, and change her avoidant or unhelpful behaviours to liberate herself from the clutches of BDD.

In Part II we will talk you through our approach and introduce you to the techniques you need to overcome body image problems and BDD. As you read through and try the exercises for yourself, you will see how you can start to change your unhelpful thinking patterns, tolerate and alleviate your difficult feelings, and modify unhelpful behaviours (including avoidance) that are likely to be dominating your life. We will give you a better understanding of your problems so that you're equipped to challenge them effectively.

The method we're going to share with you in this book is based on Cognitive Behavioural Therapy (CBT), which is a well-established, highly effective treatment approach to BDD and body dissatisfaction problems. At its heart, CBT is the study of the relationship between things that happen in your life, how you interpret them, and your physiological, emotional and behavioural responses to them. CBT can help you recognise the ways in which you think, believe and interpret events (all of which we call cognition) and then help you develop them into more helpful and adaptive ways of thinking. We aim to reduce the severity and intensity of your unpleasant emotions, and educate you on how you react physiologically to an event. Finally, we want to modify and banish unhelpful behavioural responses (both mental and physical) to these events.

CBT is the best treatment that we have to date for body image problems; it is evidence-based and it hands over the tools of treatment, recovery, and maintenance to you. Think of this approach as a toolbox – you may find some of the exercises and challenges to be very useful, others less so, but please read through the whole book before you decide which are which. It is within your reach to overcome your body image problems and BDD, so that you can build a healthier, more accepting relationship with your body and yourself.

We also believe it is important to take a compassionate approach[1] to treatment. To overcome your body dissatisfaction and BDD you need to have compassion for yourself. Compassion is defined as the feeling you get when you want to alleviate someone's suffering. In this case, that someone is you.

> In order to change, you have to take a journey that is non-judgemental and does not involve blaming yourself for your difficulties. You must be kind to yourself during your journey; you are a worthwhile person and deserve to be treated in a compassionate, warm, and supportive way, especially by yourself.

Treating yourself in a kind and non-judgemental way is incredibly important and helpful for your recovery. On your journey, there may be times when you feel that it isn't going as well as you'd hoped, or that it feels too hard. But if you treat yourself with patience and understanding, rather than criticism and blame, this will give you the courage you need to overcome such roadblocks.

People with body image problems and BDD can get better with self-guided CBT approaches like this book.[2] However, you may still want to seek one-to-one therapeutic support and advice alongside this book. In fact, if you have severe BDD we would recommend that you also seek individual therapy. If you do, please make sure you find someone who understands and has experience with Cognitive Behavioural Therapy in treating body image issues.

We ask you to embark upon reading this book with an open mind, and remember that there are many people who are struggling just like you. The fact that you're reading this book means you have taken the first step towards your recovery. In the space of a year, Chloe went from being a virtual recluse to living a considerably more fulfilling life.

We think that Chloe has been incredibly brave in opening up about her life and sharing her experience with BDD in this book. Body image problems and body dysmorphia are still so misunderstood in society. And that's one of the reasons why this book is so important. The more people who understand what BDD and body image problems are – not what the media says they are – the more our society will find ways to improve body image from an earlier age and help people suffering with BDD and body image problems to access appropriate help.

## WHAT IS BODY IMAGE?

We hear the term body image in the media a lot, but what does it actually mean?

Body image is your perception of your own physical appearance when you look at yourself in the mirror, see photos of yourself, or picture yourself in your mind's eye. Your ideas about your body image will also be influenced by what you believe other people think about your appearance.

Your body image can be positive or negative. It is dynamic and can fluctuate between being positive and negative. It can change as you mature and grow older, or in response to life experiences such as trauma or health difficulties. It can also change due to seemingly insignificant events, such as a person making a comment (which might seem trivial to others), or catching a glimpse of yourself at an unflattering angle.

We should also point out that, just because you may not like certain parts of your body or feel like you need to lose some weight, it doesn't mean that you necessarily have a body image issue. Equally, if your appearance has changed, possibly as a result of an accident, if there is something about your appearance that might be considered unusual, or you have what might be called an unconventional appearance, that does not mean that you will necessarily have body image issues either. In fact, people often celebrate these and other differences.

Body image issues are more generally associated with unhelpful thoughts that you can have about your body which cause emotional distress, including anxiety, shame, and sadness. Body image issues usually result in a series of strategies designed to modify and / or hide parts of the body.

These unhelpful thoughts can become all-consuming, and are otherwise known as "obsessions" or "preoccupations". Some people think that they will only ever be able to experience any kind of confidence or happiness if they change the way they look, and they spend countless hours thinking of ways to change, hide, or camouflage parts of their body. Sometimes they will avoid social events and public places altogether.

## POSITIVE BODY IMAGE

**People with a positive body image can:**

- Perceive their body objectively
- Appreciate their body shape and size
- Understand that appearance is only one feature of a person
- Appreciate that the appearance of their body does not say anything about their character or values
- Accept the uniqueness of their body

**People with a negative body image might:**

- Have a distorted perception of parts of their body or body shape (that is, believe that parts of their body are not as they really are)
- Believe they are ugly or unattractive
- Feel anxious or ashamed about their body
- Feel awkward and uncomfortable in their own body
- Worry constantly about their appearance and what other people think about their appearance

Your body image is influenced by your own self-observation, seeing yourself in photos, seeing your reflection in mirrors, other people's reactions to you, and how you interpret other people's reactions. It is a subjective, constructed image, reinforced by many things.

## WHAT ARE BODY IMAGE PROBLEMS?

A person with body image problems or body dissatisfaction will feel unhappy about some aspect of their appearance. They will think about their appearance a great deal and the problem will significantly interfere with their life in some way, e.g. they will feel the need to avoid specific situations including social events, relationships, or intimacy. People with body image problems usually have a distorted view of what they look like. They may feel that the size or shape of their body is a sign of failure that is clearly visible to those around them. They often compare themselves or specific features of their appearance with others. They are likely to spend a disproportionate amount of time hiding aspects of their body, fixing or masking certain features, checking how they look, and worrying about their appearance.

Of course, it is normal to dislike certain aspects of your appearance or physique. It is normal to try to look your best in certain situations or feel the need to improve your appearance. It is also normal, if you have a notable physical difference, or something considered unusual in your appearance, that you might want these to change. But things that distinguish a person with body image problems from someone with normal body dissatisfaction are:

- The amount of time they spend thinking about, trying to fix, masking or hiding their appearance or certain features

- The level of impact on their day-to-day life, and the level of distress they feel when thinking about their appearance

We know that dissatisfaction can escalate into an obsessive preoccupation with an aspect of a person's appearance. Somebody's sense of self-worth can be so strongly linked with appearance that if their body image is skewed, it will significantly undermine their sense of self-worth. When that happens, it impacts on how clever, worthy, or capable they believe they are compared with others. It can perpetuate feelings of disgust and self-loathing, leaving them feeling exposed, self-conscious in social situations, and awkward and uncomfortable in their own body.

While body image problems are common, and can vary in severity, they can also be part of a more serious mental health disorder. One of these is Body Dysmorphic Disorder (BDD or body dysmorphia), which Chloe suffered from. However, a negative body image is also present in other mental health disorders, for example eating disorders. We will briefly discuss these later in Part II, but if you suffer with an eating disorder we recommend that you seek treatment for that specific problem, which should also cover negative body image, as we won't be covering eating disorder treatment in this book.

## SO WHAT IS BODY DYSMORPHIC DISORDER?

Body Dysmorphic Disorder (BDD) is a diagnosable mental disorder, in which a person is preoccupied with a defect (often imagined) in their appearance. This preoccupation is often referred to as an "obsession". This perceived or slight defect is generally not observable, or appears very slight to others. The person suffering with BDD engages in repetitive behaviours in response to this preoccupation in order to reduce their distress, and this preoccupation also causes significant distress or problems in their life.

People with BDD perceive themselves as deeply flawed and ugly. They fixate upon a minimal or non-existent "flaw" in their appearance. For this reason, throughout the book we will use the words "perceived flaw(s)" to describe the part(s) of the body that they are preoccupied with and distressed about. Their concerns may be so severe that they shun human contact, for fear of what people will think when they see them, or in the belief that other people should be spared from seeing them altogether. The emotional impact can be devastating. Somebody suffering from BDD may have to attend events or go about everyday life under extreme duress, or may even feel compelled to withdraw from society. This leads to isolation.

It is impossible for people who suffer with BDD to believe that anyone who says nice or even neutral things about their appearance is telling the truth. In their worldview, it makes more sense to believe that those people are being kind, or lying, to try to save their feelings.

Some common BDD obsessions relate to the eyes, nose, skin, chin, lips, and neck. When we talk about obsessions, we mean things that completely occupy the mind for the majority of a person's day-to-day life. People suffering with BDD can fixate on one or multiple aspects of their appearance. The flaws they see may be very subtle (e.g.

one ear may appear slightly bigger than the other), or imagined altogether (e.g. they may believe that they have an unusually large nose, when objective observers believe that their nose is average size or smaller).

It is important to know that BDD is not a vanity issue, and people with BDD aren't usually obsessed with being perfect. It is an obsessional disorder, and people become fixated on trying to change their appearance and feel normal. Life as somebody suffering with BDD can be extremely lonely. People with BDD may try to avoid social situations altogether, or else they will expend vast amounts of effort just to function in society.

Living a "normal" life can be inordinately difficult for people suffering with BDD. Even if they have a normal routine involving school, college, or work, their overriding concerns about their appearance can cloud everything else. Somebody with BDD may be so preoccupied with their perceived flaw or trying to find ways to minimise how noticeable it is, that their focus on other tasks is diminished.

BDD is associated with a number of obsessive compulsive behaviours. These are the repetitive behaviours we mentioned before, which a person may feel compelled to do in an effort to minimise the likelihood of the flaw (perceived or real) being noticed, and to ensure that other people don't get offended by their appearance. These behaviours include, but are not limited to:

• Checking appearance as often as possible, either by touch or in a mirror, or
• Avoiding any mirrors or reflective surfaces, as they remind them of their appearance and thus cause extreme anxiety

- Reassurance seeking – asking people to provide reassurance that a perceived or small flaw is not too visible, or has not worsened
- Skin picking in an effort to remove perceived flaws
- Excessive grooming
- Frequently comparing appearance with others, online or in person
- Avoiding situations that may draw attention to their appearance. This will include avoidance of photographs, social events and intimacy
- Attempts to correct, camouflage, or cover up the perceived flaw. This can even go so far as getting surgery to "correct" the problem
- Scanning the internet and gathering data on their perceived flaw and possible solutions that can "fix" the problem

## ISN'T A PREOCCUPATION WITH APPEARANCE THE SAME AS VANITY?

One of the sad things about many people we see who experience BDD is that they have refused to consider treatment for so long. Why? Simply because society has taught them that body dissatisfaction is the result of excessive vanity. It isn't. People who have BDD aren't usually seeking perfection. Most are not trying to be flawlessly beautiful. They are just looking to be acceptable, so that they can walk to the shop without offending people who, they believe, shouldn't have to look at them. They are simply trying to reach a point where they look "normal" enough to fit into society.

Although these issues occur in BDD most prominently, they are common in people with all body image problems. It is often the degree of severity and the impact on everyday life that differentiates the two. We discuss this more in Part II Section 3. However, the treatment techniques and experiments we will suggest in Part II will help with both BDD and body image problems.

## THE BELIEFS BEHIND
## BODY DISSATISFACTION AND BDD

Every person with body dissatisfaction and BDD believes there is an obvious problem with their body and their appearance, even though to an objective observer, these problems are not noticeable or significant. So how can people with body dissatisfaction believe one thing, while others believe something so different?

Well, a belief is not an objective thought. Rather, our beliefs about ourselves and our appearance are made up of a combination of our experiences, ideas, assumptions, and thoughts. They are subjective and personal.

For example, someone with body image issues might see someone glance at them briefly in the street. As a result, they might then assume that they were being stared at because of an issue with their appearance. This belief causes them to quickly hide away and avoid going out as much as possible. Sometimes a casual, fleeting comment from a friend or family member can feed a person's growing belief that they have a physical deformity. Or, very much like we will hear later from Chloe, an unpleasant encounter or experience with someone could lead a person to believe they are inferior, and this then seeps into beliefs about their own appearance. To be clear, these kinds of beliefs don't form overnight. The initial idea that there is an issue with your appearance gains strength over time – and in the next chapter, we'll tell you a story, demonstrating how ideas turn into assumptions which then become entrenched beliefs.

## WHAT IS ANXIETY?

When discussing body image issues, we talk a lot about anxiety.

We've all felt anxiety, whether during entering an exam, or plucking up the courage to speak to someone we like. If you've ever thought you were going to be late for a meeting, you'll have experienced the intensity of anxiety as you become later and later for your appointment. But then the feelings will fade as you finally arrive, or you manage to make your excuses.

Severe anxiety is different; it can manifest itself as a diagnosable mental disorder, such as panic disorder, or it can be a prominent feature of another mental condition, such as Body Dysmorphic Disorder.

## WHAT CAUSES ANXIETY?

Anxiety occurs when we believe we're facing a threat of some kind. Our adrenaline surges and our bodies go into fight, flight, or freeze mode. This is so that we can either stand our ground against the thing that is threatening us, run away, or freeze and play dead. This instinct goes right back to the earliest days of humanity, and it helped our caveman ancestors survive in a hostile world. It was actually a very effective inbuilt defence system.

Although it may sound strange, it's important to note that anxiety isn't trying to harm you. It's actually trying to look after you. The problem is that we live in a very different world to the cavemen, and we experience different kinds of threats. Nevertheless, we still get those big surges of anxiety-fuelled adrenaline that equips us to fight, freeze, or flee. The problem with anxiety occurs when we get a big adrenaline surge even though the threat we think we're facing isn't real, or is much smaller than we imagined.

## EXPERIENCING DEPRESSION AS A RESULT OF BODY IMAGE PROBLEMS AND BDD

Unsurprisingly, people who suffer with body image problems and BDD often experience depression as a result. If you have body image issues or BDD, then it can occupy your thoughts for a lot of your waking life. It is exhausting, even without all the grooming and checking you may have to do before you can even leave the house. Or perhaps you already avoid people and new situations? You may even have stopped doing the things that you used to enjoy. Experiencing less enjoyment from activities you used to enjoy is a common feature of depression, and naturally can cause you to feel down.

If you are also suffering from depression, it is important to identify which came first – your body image issues or your depression. If you were clinically depressed before the onset of body image issues or BDD, then you may need treatment for the depression first. This might be a combination of medication and psychological therapy. But if depression followed after the onset of your body image issues or BDD, then it may lessen as you treat these problems.

If you do worry that the depression has been with you longer than your other problems, or is so entrenched it might prevent you from being able to benefit from this help, then we do suggest you see your doctor to discuss further treatment options for depression. We talk more about dealing with depression in Part II Section 1.

## DEALING WITH THOUGHTS ABOUT ENDING YOUR LIFE

If you have experienced thoughts about suicide, believe you don't deserve to live any longer, or have already made plans to end your life, please let someone know immediately. You can speak to a friend, relative, or your doctor, and they will support you through the next steps. It is important to seek help immediately, and you can always return to this treatment book once those suicidal thoughts have abated. You can also find more help and advice about suicidal thoughts at www.shawmindfoundation.org.

## GIVE YOURSELF TIME

Just a final thought, before we continue with Chloe's story … We understand that you will want to recover from your body image issues or BDD as soon as possible, but we just ask that you give yourself some time to enact the strategies you will learn in this book. While we can't promise that a full recovery will happen immediately, we can tell you that by using the methods we describe in Part II, you will start to see improvements quickly. However, for a sustained recovery and a more positive approach to your body and appearance, you will need to continue to use these strategies after your initial success and achievements, to ensure that the positive changes really do become embedded into your daily life.

Inspired by Chloe's story and with our help, you are about to start your journey towards a new acceptance of your body and appearance.

# PART I
## CHLOE'S STORY

# CHAPTER 1

# A DEATH IN THE FAMILY

 ***Chloe:*** Was I always likely to have BDD? How can you tell?

If you'd have had to pick someone out of a line-up as the child that was going to develop body dysmorphia, would you have chosen me?

I was 3lb 4oz (1.4kg) when I was born – so small that a natural birth would have been dangerous, so Mum had to have a caesarean. Afterwards, she couldn't feed me, so they had to put a tube up my nose, which, looking back at the videos, it's clear I wasn't too fond of. My twin, Olivia, was about 5lbs and we were born on our mum's birthday.

We had a great start in life. You really couldn't ask for kinder, more supportive parents. And we always knew they wanted the best for us. As children we were always encouraged to experience lots of different things, so I got to play the violin, try golf, and enjoy singing and acting.

All my early memories are warm, happy ones. I think my earliest memory is being in the kitchen with my grandma when we were three years old. She was trying to hold on to us, and we were running around the kitchen, laughing.

I certainly credit a lot of the things I like about myself to Mum, Dad and my grandparents. They're the sort of people I aspire to be. I know how lucky I've been to have their love and support, especially as my life became more difficult. And there was always Olivia. Because of her, I never felt scared of starting anything new because I knew she'd be there right alongside me. Until I met Lauren and Annemarie, she was the only person to whom I could really talk about what I was going through.

People think it must be annoying for me to have to share my birthday with my twin, but I've really never minded that. I don't like being the centre of attention, so it worked well for me. When people sing happy birthday, it just feels like the most awkward moment, so it's good to be able to share that attention with another person. I never know what to do with myself in that situation. I cringe and my toes curl with embarrassment.

Growing up, we were always a little bit different physically. When we got to the age of seven, I was quite slim and tomboyish and Olivia was slightly bigger than me. We never knew why, because we ate exactly the same things and did all the same activities. Even though no one said anything to Olivia about her weight, I was aware of her being a little larger than other girls our age and I was always slightly protective towards her because of it. I definitely didn't want anyone saying anything to her because I knew it wasn't her fault.

I suppose that was my first awareness of body image. Instinctively I seemed to know that people could be unkind about appearance, even if they didn't necessarily mean to be. When we were seven or eight, we were having a meal in a restaurant. Olivia had a starter, a main course, and a dessert. There was an American man at another table, who looked over at my sister. He said to her, in a very jolly way and without any kind of malice, 'Do you have a cupboard under there?' We all laughed, but at the same time I thought, *Why is he thinking that?*

I think that was the only time anyone said anything about her weight, but something clicked. It felt wrong. She was my sister and she didn't deserve that. Perhaps it was just my own oversensitivity creeping in – but I kept thinking about how that incident would have affected me. Hearing a comment like that really brought home to me just how obsessed with appearance people are.

I feel enormous empathy for people and I've always been that way. I was aware of feeling more protective of Olivia when we were around boys. (Whether she needed me to be or not!) We came from an all-girls school, so if we did a half-term activity, I was suddenly aware of that whole boys / girls divide. It seemed to me that boys were crueler than girls. I don't remember anyone saying anything to my sister, but again, I think boys just made me feel warier, as if I was on alert.

I needn't have worried. Olivia always coped with whatever life threw at her. And now, she's engaged to be married. I'm really happy for her, but at the same time, it feels like the end of an era and I'm still waiting to see how our relationship will evolve. I still confide in her. I still see her as often as I can. But she's moving on with her life, while I feel like I'm left behind. That's not her fault. It's not anyone's fault. It's just the way things are. We went along the same path for so long, but I suppose she carried on growing up while I got stuck.

Physically, we're a similar height and weight now, so it's quite hard to tell us apart. But temperamentally and emotionally, we're quite different. Olivia gets more riled about things and she really knows how to let off steam after a bad day at work, whereas I internalise everything. I've never found it easy to let things out. Perhaps if I'd been able to – perhaps if I hadn't lived in my head for so long – things might have been different. I don't know.

I was a secure, happy child though. At primary school, I always felt like I did my best, and that gave me a strong sense of self-worth. I felt like I was following the values set for me by my mum and dad, and I felt content with my place in the world. I sang in the school choir and I loved acting. I even got a big part in the Year 6 leaving play, *Annie*. I had to sing, solo, in front of a crowd. And I loved it! I couldn't possibly imagine doing that now.

I don't remember looking in the mirror as a child. I know I must have done, but I don't remember having any strong reactions to the face I saw looking back at me. I didn't have a very clear sense of how I looked. Even in secondary school, there didn't seem to be quite as much value put on appearance compared to today. There were people at school who would say, 'Oh, this person's ugly ...' but it wasn't like nowadays; now everything is on social media. Back then, people weren't so defined by their appearance.

I didn't really look at photos much when I was growing up, but I would sometimes look back at pictures of me as a young child. To start with, I didn't even have a problem with having school photos taken. I wasn't desperate to go and get them developed, but I saw them as a nice keepsake of a time in my life, nothing more.

It all sounds very normal, doesn't it? We lived in a normal house, and my mum and dad had pretty average incomes, although they managed to send us to a private school, rather than a state school. Most of the people we went to school with had horses and tennis courts and everything they ever wanted. My best friend at primary school lived next door to Ringo Starr, one of The Beatles! I wasn't intimidated though. It sounds so weird now, but I was mostly outgoing. In fact, I really loved primary school. We were the normal kids in a school full of super-rich girls, and yet I don't ever remember feeling out of place. I was totally comfortable in my own skin.

I do have one unpleasant memory from primary school, and the way I felt has stayed with me ever since ... When I was about eight years old, I was trying really hard to please my teacher. She asked a question about the Romans and, because I liked history, I put my hand up, and I did that slightly stupid thing of waving it about a bit. I wasn't going over the top, but I really wanted to answer! And she just looked at me and said, 'Yeah, we know you know,' and the way she said it really affected me. I know that teachers are supposed to be more inclusive, but no one else had their hand up, so I was really taken aback. At that moment, I wondered if perhaps it wasn't really worth trying quite so hard. It may not sound like much, but as I was aged eight or nine, I think this was the first blow to my self-confidence.

A couple of years later, I remember Olivia knocking over a water cup by accident when we were painting, and the teacher just went mad at her. It was so unpleasant because my sister really liked the teacher and always did everything she could to please her. In my mind, I was shouting at the teacher, 'What do you think you're doing? She didn't do it on purpose!' I was so upset for Olivia. This person that my sister really liked was berating her for the smallest of things.

These things always stuck with me. They changed the way I thought – the teachers dampened my enthusiasm. I was always wary after that. I knew then that life could be really unfair.

While most of our primary school friends continued in private education, Mum and Dad couldn't afford to continue paying for secondary schooling, so we moved to a state school. When I was 10, my class had fewer than 15 people in it, but when I moved to secondary school, there were over 30 of us. It was quite a shock to the system.

I really wanted to be in the same class as Olivia in secondary school, but they kept us apart. I only knew two other girls in my year – one from my primary school, and one from my nursery school, but they weren't in any of my classes, so I felt like I didn't know anyone.

As soon as my new classmates found out what school I was from, they thought I was the poshest person they'd ever met. They assumed I came from a wealthy family and thought I must be an incredibly brainy, straight-A student. In our first music lesson, we had to take it in turns to say if we'd played a musical instrument before. Although I'd already given it up, I'd played the oboe in my final years at primary school. When I said it, everyone looked at me as if I'd said something in Chinese!

Being in a private school is like being in a bubble. You don't really see the other side of things. So moving to a state secondary school was eye-opening, but in a good way. We'd always been comfortable. My family wasn't rich, but we weren't poor either. So I reflected that it was good to have this experience. I may not have liked secondary school, but I'm grateful for the broader insight it gave me.

At first, it felt like such an alien environment. I felt very distant from the teachers, and from a lot of the students as well. In primary school, I had been keen to volunteer for extra work and always put my hand up, but I very quickly learnt that you don't do that in secondary school. Not unless you want people to make fun of you. So when the teacher said, 'Hands up!' I'd fight the urge and say the answer in my head instead. It felt like I was still answering, without actually being ridiculed for doing it. So it took me a while to settle, and it took everyone else a while to realise I wasn't this rich girl who was incredibly smart. I just tried to do what you're "supposed" to do: have friends, do my work, socialise – but I wasn't really enjoying any of it. I was simply going through the motions.

Up until about age 13, I also attended stage school and at first I really enjoyed it. We did singing, acting, and dancing. This was the first time I noticed I enjoyed doing things more in a group than individually, but it was also one of the first times I started feeling really, consistently, self-conscious. There were some good dancers there, and I started comparing myself with them. I knew I wasn't the best dancer, so I always ended up at the back of the group. Clearly my habit of comparing myself unfavourably with others was starting to take hold.

The problem was, I knew I wasn't getting better at dancing, and there wasn't anything I could do about it. It wasn't like maths, where I could take up extra tuition (I really struggled with maths and hated how I felt when I got bad results on my tests). But singing and dancing were different. I kept wondering how I could make myself better, but I couldn't really give myself a better singing voice, and my acting and dancing weren't improving no matter how hard I tried. So I started to become more and more uncomfortable with myself, and started losing faith in my abilities.

This was also the first time I started avoiding situations and retreating from doing the things I liked. Slowly but surely, I began to miss dancing events deliberately. For instance, when we had to do monologues and duets, I wasn't comfortable with the thought of it, so I just didn't turn up!

I was becoming less secure in my own skin. I didn't know how to cope with being bad at certain subjects and I didn't feel like I could ask the teachers for help. There was a real range of people in my form including some very sporty people and some very arty people. I started comparing myself with them too. I'd try to learn from them – I'd watch what they did and try to practise their techniques over and over again. But it just didn't work. I knew I couldn't be good at everything, but I just wanted to be okay. And when I felt like I wasn't, those feelings of inadequacy started to take over, and I wanted to hide myself away.

Any little illness became the catalyst for time off school. I knew my grades were good enough for me to pull through, but Mum knew something was wrong. I just wasn't sure what to tell her.

By the time I was 14, my social group had changed too. The friends I'd made in the first couple of years left for a different school, went to a different form, or moved into different friendship groups. So I was stuck in the middle with another group of people who didn't really fit anywhere else. We weren't popular, and we weren't unpopular; we were in no man's land. The older I got, the more I realised they weren't proper friends. I worked hard to please them – I would be the one to invite them round and buy them pizza and presents. But that wasn't the basis of proper friendships. It was more a case of me saying, 'Like me! Please!'

I knew that everyone talked about everyone else behind their back, and I was desperate not to be included in the endless round of rumours. I wanted to keep my head down and not be noticed, so I thought that if I worked hard to please everyone, maybe people wouldn't talk about me.

My attitude to school was changing. I thought about that incident with the teacher at primary school a lot. And suddenly it made sense. Maybe she'd been right. What was the point in being enthusiastic about anything if it meant that people were just going to make fun of me? It wasn't cool to be interested in anything. It wasn't cool to do well or get good grades.

If you'd compared me and my sister at that time, you'd have seen a big difference. She was visibly more outgoing and sociable than I was. I felt as if things were changing. My perception of the world was shifting and life was getting harder. But looking back, I can see that I was still at the top of the spiral, and things were never going to be the same again …

In 2009, aged 16, I was in my last year of secondary school and working hard on my GCSEs. That's when my grandma died. Because we were such a close-knit family, her death hit us all really hard. Grandma and Grandad's house was our hub – a halfway point for everyone in our family. So much of my childhood is bound up in memories of happy days playing in their garden, magical Christmases, and wonderful dinners.

In fact, everyone loved Grandma. She was just one of the nicest people you could meet; so warm and welcoming. She was like the head of our family, and everyone just gravitated towards her. Along with Mum, she taught me so much, even little things like how to eat soup properly! I remember when Grandad was doing it wrong – putting his head to the bowl – and she was saying, 'No Grandad, you bring your spoon to your mouth!' It was so funny.

I cherish those memories of the person Grandma really was. Even now, the smell of her perfume brings back so many happy memories. But she changed a lot in the last year of her life. Her mental state deteriorated rapidly because of her dementia. It started off with little things, like forgetting dates and getting names wrong – so she'd confuse my mum and my aunt, and me and my sister, little things like that. But it got worse and worse. She started to talk about the old days more and more and she confused the past with the present. She'd show me pictures and identify people wrongly, but even when we pointed out her mistake, she wouldn't hear it.

One of the saddest things was when my grandparents argued. It was almost like Grandad was trying to snap her out of it. He understood what was happening, but he was still frustrated. I'd never seen them argue about anything before.

My mum and aunt decided it was best to get a live-in carer, because Grandad had never done any cleaning or anything like that in his whole life! And of course he was finding it hard too; the love of his life was fading away before his eyes. The carer we brought in was a lovely lady, but Grandma really resented her. It got to the stage where she became quite rude – and she was never normally rude about anything or anyone. The person she was turning into was so unlike the warm, caring person we knew. It was hard to take.

In February 2009, we went to my grandparents' house for the weekend while the carer was away. I didn't want Mum to go on her own because I knew how sad and stressful it could be, so I suggested that Mum spend some time with Grandad while I sat with Grandma. For the first time in a long time, everything felt normal. Grandma seemed more like her old self. I remember we sat and watched *Dad's Army* and we just laughed and talked. And then a trailer came on for *Who Do You Think You Are?* – the programme where they trace people's ancestors – and she used to really enjoy watching that, so we just chatted about it. Then we said good night. It was so weird because she suddenly seemed just like she used to be. The next morning she came into the room I was staying in and drew back the curtains, just like she used to when I was a little girl. It was so wonderfully normal.

After we talked a bit, she went downstairs to join Mum. I was just getting dressed when I heard Mum shouting ...

I don't remember racing down the stairs. I just remember seeing Grandma on the kitchen floor. I thought she must have fallen out of her chair, but she'd had a stroke. Mum was already phoning the ambulance, so I just sat on the floor with Grandma and held her. For a long time afterwards, I thought that maybe I should have done something differently. I don't know what ... maybe I could have held her differently, or done something ... But I was on autopilot, so I just sat there with her while Mum organised everything. I remember thinking that I had to be the one to sit with Grandma – that Mum shouldn't have to see her like that.

I went to visit her in hospital, but it was so difficult. I didn't want that to be the last image I had of her. I wanted my abiding memory to be when she came into my room on that last morning when, just for a few moments, everything felt so normal.

Grandma died about a week later. It felt like the end of an era. And I suppose that in retrospect, it was the beginning of the fall for me. After she died, I retreated into myself and became more and more withdrawn. Very slowly I stopped turning up for school – a day or two here and there to start with, and then more. I just didn't want to go back. Eventually it got to a stage where Mum or Dad would have to encourage me.

I couldn't talk about what had happened with anyone. I couldn't trust my friends to understand what I was going through. How could they? I couldn't talk to my family either. It hadn't been them down there on the floor with Grandma. It had been me, so I felt like I couldn't really share the pain of my experience with anyone, not even Mum. Not even Olivia. That was the first time in my life that I felt really isolated.

Everything changed without Grandma. But of course, it wasn't just my loss. I tried to imagine what it was like for Grandad. It changed him. You could see it in his eyes. They'd been together for more than 50 years, and she had loved looking after him, so I could see how lonely he was. It must have been awful to lose half your life like that – they had been like two parts of the same person.

We tried to carry on as normal, because we knew it was what Grandma would have wanted. So we did the same things and kept the same routines. But it felt empty without Grandma. It was almost as if there was an empty chair in the room with a spotlight on it.

At school I was just about doing enough to get me through. I knew how to coast. But in every other respect, I was struggling. My grief was turning into depression, and everything else started to spiral from there. Bit by bit, I was changing – backing away from normal life, avoiding school, shunning friends and withdrawing from the world. I was feeling very low, which worried me.

I sensed that I was different in some way from my peers. At this point, I wasn't aware of body dysmorphia at all, but looking back, I can see that my preoccupation with my appearance was slowly emerging, and my worries about what other people thought about me were becoming stronger.

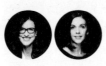

***Lauren and Annemarie:*** Reading this chapter shows you just how self-conscious Chloe was becoming. It happened as she was becoming more aware of how she might be judged by people, and how her appearance could be assessed by others. At the same time as this growing awareness, Chloe experienced a significant life event – the loss of a beloved relative. As her depression deepened, it made her increasingly vulnerable to BDD.

## DEALING WITH LOSS AND GUILT

Chloe clearly had a very close bond with her grandmother, and her passing was the loss of a significant attachment figure – as well as someone who accepted Chloe unreservedly for who she was. Unconditional love is very precious, and as Chloe was learning to deal with the loss of her grandmother, she was also learning that in her peer group at school, there were many conditions to being liked. It was the opposite of her relationship with her grandmother.

One of the things that made her grandmother's passing more difficult was that Chloe experienced so much guilt. She mentions that she wishes she could have held her grandmother differently after she collapsed in her home, even though it was clear there was nothing else she could have done.

Chloe didn't know how to deal with her feelings, and she was aware that her family was suffering too. For that reason – and because her particular experience of the event had been different to theirs – she didn't feel able to talk about it with them, or with anyone else. She explains that she couldn't confide in her friends. The result was that she had to try to deal with her grief completely on her own. That is a heavy burden for anyone, and it came at a point in her life when she was not so confident of her place in life. She was unhappy at school, had less than stable friendship groups and was becoming increasingly depressed.

## DEPRESSION, BODY IMAGE ISSUES, AND BDD

It's easy to see the link between body image issues, BDD, and depression. If your life is being dominated by worries over your appearance, then it is going to have a profound impact on your mood. And then the low mood makes you more vulnerable to unhelpful thinking patterns and behaviours. For example, people who experience BDD or body dissatisfaction can feel like their lives are restricted due to worries about their appearance, and as a consequence they start avoiding people, places, and situations. The longer this goes on, the less likely they are to experience the same simple pleasures as other people, or feel that they are achieving anything, and that just results in further depression.

Depression often results in low motivation levels and lethargy and this makes it hard for people to leave the house and try to do anything fun or productive. Of course this makes the depression worse, which makes the unhelpful thinking worse and so on ... In addition, if you've got strong critical beliefs about any part of yourself, they will inevitably contribute to a low mood. So you can see how the mix of BDD, body image problems, and depression becomes a vicious cycle which is difficult to break.

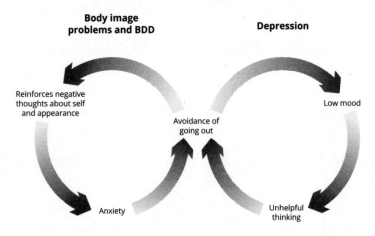

*Figure 1:* *The interaction of depression and body image problems.*

Between the bouts of BDD, severe body image problems, and depression, people's lives can stall. And this is one of the big problems for people in recovery as they find that they skip big parts of normal development as a side effect of their issues. Other people their age might be out socialising, dating, studying, or working. They are constantly interacting with people, finding their social norms, and building social confidence. But people who are crippled by depression, BDD, and severe body image problems don't get to do that. They don't get to socially experiment like other people do, and therefore don't build any social confidence or independence.

The same is true for people experiencing milder body image issues. By their late teens, they won't have the same social experience and skills as other people; they might not even have the same career opportunities. So already there are lots of things that can inspire or exacerbate depression.

## SYMPTOMS OF DEPRESSION

Here is a checklist of some of the signs that may indicate you are depressed:[3]

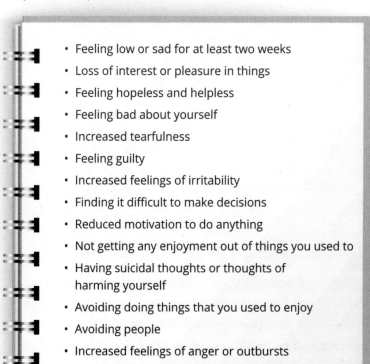

- Feeling low or sad for at least two weeks
- Loss of interest or pleasure in things
- Feeling hopeless and helpless
- Feeling bad about yourself
- Increased tearfulness
- Feeling guilty
- Increased feelings of irritability
- Finding it difficult to make decisions
- Reduced motivation to do anything
- Not getting any enjoyment out of things you used to
- Having suicidal thoughts or thoughts of harming yourself
- Avoiding doing things that you used to enjoy
- Avoiding people
- Increased feelings of anger or outbursts

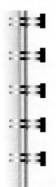

- Moving or speaking more slowly than usual
- Increase or decrease in appetite or weight
- Unexplained aches and pains
- Disturbed sleep (for example, finding it hard to fall asleep at night or waking up very early in the morning) or sleeping more than you need (adults need on average between six and eight hours a night).

If you've identified that you are suffering from five of these symptoms, one of which must be low mood or sadness, or loss of interest or pleasure, and you've felt like this for the last two weeks or longer, then it is likely that you are also suffering from depression.

If you have a history of clinical depression before you developed BDD or body image problems, or if it is so severe that you think it will prevent you from recovering from your body image problems or BDD, you should consider having treatment for the depression first. This would probably involve a combination of therapy and anti-depressant drugs. This will help put you in a better place to start tackling your BDD and body image problems.

Why? The techniques we use to help control and treat the BDD and body image concerns will also have a positive effect on your depression and, over time, may reduce or eliminate your depression altogether. However, if you're struggling to untangle the order of events, a psychologist can help you determine which came first, and help you determine the best next steps to take.

The checklist above will help you to identify whether you're suffering from depression, and in our treatment programme in Part II, we'll look at the issue of depression in more detail. However, if you've been having these symptoms for a long time, and you're finding it difficult to get up in the morning because of them, please do seek help or advice from your doctor.

At the beginning of the book, Chloe said that at her lowest point, she wondered if she could go on living. At that time, Chloe had almost given up. She was alone and afraid. She didn't know what was happening to her. She didn't know if what she was experiencing was normal, or if it would pass, or if there was anyone else like her. She had little or no hope of anything changing.

I'd just like to add that if you are having serious thoughts about ending your life (and the thought of dying no longer scares you), you have already made plans to end your life, or you've carried out a suicide attempt before, please seek professional help now. You are reading this book. That is a great sign that on some level, no matter how deep down, you believe (or just hope) that things can improve. You want to live, just not in the way you're living now. If, at any time, you feel you're in real danger of attempting to end your life, please ask for help. You can also visit: www.shawmindfoundation.org for more help and information.

## CHAPTER 2

## WITHDRAWING FROM THE WORLD

*Chloe:* I was becoming increasingly socially withdrawn. But looking back, I can see that it didn't really start when my grandma got ill. Even before that, I remember times when my grandparents came to our house and I would stay in my room instead of going down to see them. Still to this day, I don't know why I did that. It wasn't that I didn't want to see them. But I felt, emotionally and physically, like I couldn't leave my room – as if there was something stopping me.

Little did I know then that it was the start of something awful. I wasn't very socially anxious at the time, despite the odd bit of nervousness when meeting new people. And so it was weird and frustrating and confusing, because I loved spending time with my grandparents. I only wish I'd spent more time with them before they passed away.

As I was pulling away from external life, my school friends were starting to document more of their day-to-day life online. I looked at the pictures. Everyone looked at the pictures. But the more I looked, the worse I felt.

I started comparing myself with three girls in particular, and I wondered how I could make myself look more like them. They had long hair, their make-up was really nice and they looked effortlessly pretty. In my mind, they were the ideal, but I felt inferior to everyone. It was all about appearance. I didn't compare myself with them in terms of academic achievement, or our interests, or anything else.

It affected everything. So when I went swimming with friends, all I could think about was the dreaded moment when we'd reveal our swimming costumes. Before we went, I stood in front of the mirror, pulling back the small bit of fat on my hips so I could see what I would look like without it. Then I'd try to find the best way to hold in my stomach, and the best angle for people to look at me so I would know how I had to stand. And I would do that for half an hour at a time. I was so paranoid about the tops of my thighs; I felt like a beached whale. Being surrounded by so many skinny friends really didn't help, it just added to my paranoid thinking.

Physical education lessons were a nightmare, especially in the changing room before and after. I used to change out of my clothes at the speed of lightning, just in case anyone saw my shameful body. It was always a horrible, humiliating experience.

Shopping became another big issue, and eventually I stopped buying clothes altogether. I knew nothing would suit me, and seeing myself from all angles in a well-lit changing room was utter hell. I was becoming completely fixated on my appearance. I didn't know if the feelings I were having were normal for a girl my age, or if this was something else.

It had started with weight, but more and more, I was fixating on my face and my neck. I was starting to notice all my flaws and the bad skin and the ugliness ...

I started to dread having my photo taken. School photo day got more difficult as the years went on, especially when I was around 14 or 15. I always tried to be sick on those days, but Mum was wise to me, and always encouraged me to go in. I remember cringing and blushing through the whole painful process. My palms would get sweatier as it got closer to my turn, the butterflies would start, and I would feel more and more nauseated.

My friends were spending more and more time online, documenting every part of their daily lives. I didn't like the thought of people I didn't know seeing photos of me. If I wasn't happy with the images of myself, what on earth were they going to think? If I couldn't stay out of photos, I would spend hours scrutinising every image of myself, while comparing myself negatively against my friends' pictures.

At the end of Year 11 when I was 16, we had Prom: it was stressful enough looking for a dress, but thinking about all the photos that were going to be taken was even worse. I knew they were going to be all over social media and I wouldn't have any control over what photos would be taken, or who would share them. And, of course, this was before the days of face-tuning apps and things like that, so there was no way of controlling or enhancing what went up. Inevitably, friends always chose the most flattering shots of themselves; they didn't worry about anyone else. So it didn't matter to them if they published a rubbish photo of me so long as they looked good in it.

Still eager to please, I invited my group of friends over to our house and their parents came over to take photos. One dad even brought his high-quality camera over and was sitting on the floor to take "proper" pictures. Some girls were wearing hair extensions and I thought they looked really good, so I was starting to feel more and more insecure, and the endless photos only made it worse.

I knew that Mum would have been upset if I didn't enjoy Prom, so of course I told her it was okay. Looking back at the photos now, I don't mind them too much. But at the time, I couldn't stop scrutinising them. I spent hours reviewing them, comparing myself with everyone else in the picture, and trying to find some aspect in them that I was comfortable with. I never managed.

The thought that the photos were all out there and easily available for anyone and everyone to judge was really distressing. Every photo felt like more objective evidence of my ugliness. I was feeling more and more unhappy in my own skin, and I wanted to shut myself away.

Having talked about it with Lauren and Annemarie, I now know that I had started ruminating. I was dwelling on every little issue, holding on to it, turning it over and over in my mind, examining it from all the worst possible angles. I spent hours replaying what had happened to me and wondering what the people I had been with were really thinking of me when they looked at me. I constantly asked my mum if I looked okay.

Towards the end of secondary school at age 16, I started to retreat more and more. I went to school as little as possible and stopped spending time with my friends.

In truth, they were just people I used to see every day. We didn't connect on a deeper level. And I was tired of pretending to like the things they liked to try to fit in.

I was just about able to focus enough energy on passing my exams. I knew that if I didn't manage to do that, I wouldn't know what else to do with my life. Leaving school was a relief. I didn't have to see anyone any more, and I didn't have to worry about anyone seeing me. But I knew it couldn't last for ever. At 16, I went to college to start my A Levels. It was daunting starting all over again.

I tried to do the things you have to do to fit in. So just before October half term, I went on a trip to Alton Towers (a theme park in England) with a group from college. Everyone else was excited and taking lots of pictures. Even though I said I didn't want any photos because I knew they'd end up online, two of the girls kept trying. It was so annoying after I'd asked them nicely not to. They were trying from all angles, but I had good reflexes and was used to putting my hands up over my face so they couldn't get a proper shot. I was already feeling really vulnerable; Grandad had had a fall and gone into hospital, so I was nervous about being away from home while he was there.

When I rang home to find out how he was, all the sadness welled up inside me. I was crying and no one seemed to care. I just felt so removed from the social group. There was just one girl who came and asked if I was okay. I just wanted to go home; I wanted to be with him.

When we got to the hotel, everyone was rushing in and out of each other's rooms, and I just wanted to be on my own. There were six or seven of us in a small room, and I desperately wanted everyone to go away and leave me alone.

That half term I told Mum I didn't want to go back to college. She tried to persuade me to return. The school even said I could change my subjects, but I really didn't want to go back. I couldn't.

In the days and weeks that followed, I kept to myself, only venturing out if I really had to. I was becoming more afraid of being seen. I remember bumping into one of the girls in town who wondered where I'd been, so I just made some excuses about not being very well. The Vice Principal suggested taking a year out, and offered me counselling, but I didn't take it. I stayed at home and didn't really do anything.

Mum and Dad were worried. They assumed I was still struggling to deal with the grief. A few weeks after he had gone into hospital, Grandad died. It was eight months after Grandma's death. I hadn't gone in to see him. I couldn't. I didn't want to be selfish, but I was afraid of seeing an image of him that I couldn't get rid of. And that made me think about all the times I hadn't gone downstairs to see them when they'd visited. After that, the grief and the guilt kept on snowballing, and triggered a massive avalanche of negative emotions. I couldn't cope with it at all.

Afterwards, when people saw me, they'd innocently ask what I was up to, and I'd want to say, 'Well, my grandparents have died, so, not a lot.' I felt like I couldn't talk about it because I didn't want anyone to get upset. And I thought if it was that hard for me, what was it like for my aunt or my mum?

Mum was well into her fifties when Grandma died, so I knew that she'd been able to enjoy a good long relationship with her mum. I started worrying that I wouldn't have that luxury with my own parents. It was a morbid moment.

Mum thought I was struggling to let go of the grief, and suggested I should see a doctor, but I couldn't face it. I couldn't face anything any more. I felt like I had nothing to lose, and nothing to gain.

That was the breaking point. Basically, I stayed in my bed for about a month. Mum and Dad didn't put any pressure on me. I think perhaps they were a bit sad that I didn't do my A Levels, but they understood that it just wasn't possible. Instead, they suggested that if I wasn't going to go to college any more, then I should think about getting a part-time job. So I did it to please them. I applied for a few things – nothing I really wanted to do – and then got a job at the local McDonald's.

It took me a little while to remember everything on the tills, but that wasn't the hardest part. Every lunchtime, people from college would start drifting in. They all wanted to know what I was doing and when I was coming back, but I couldn't give them any answers. It was horrible.

I lasted three weeks at that job. After that, I fell back into the same routine. I spent as much time asleep as I could, because when you're asleep, you don't have to think about anything. I'd had to deal with two family deaths in such a short space of time, and I guess I didn't know how to react. I didn't even know if the way I was feeling was normal. I didn't know it at the time, but later I found out that the deaths exacerbated my underlying depression and emerging BDD.

I only knew that my life felt "wrong". I knew I wasn't like other people my age. But I didn't know why. It was the grief, wasn't it? It had to be. What else could it be?

 ***Lauren and Annemarie:*** Where does our awareness of our appearance come from?

Every child goes through a psychological development phase when they become self-aware and develop self-consciousness. You can see it in little things, like when a small child smiles when they see someone they like, or when they first exhibit symptoms of embarrassment or pride.[4]

If you look at a young child in front of a mirror, you will notice that before they have any sense of their own identity, they will find the whole experience funny and entertaining. They love to see how the image in the mirror replicates what they do. But as they get older and start to develop a sense of self, the experience changes. Suddenly they become shy about seeing their reflection – as if the experience of seeing how they present to the world is embarrassing.

As children grow up, their sense of self – and their sense of their appearance – will continue to evolve. A mix of comments from family and friends about their own appearance, and their impressions of other people's appearance, will impact on what they see and think when they look in the mirror.

All of this reinforces the belief that appearance is important. It is frequently commented on. The young child will hear comments like, 'Oh, what a pretty girl you are,' or 'Didn't he look smart today?' In the same way that they come to recognise good manners as a desirable trait, or understand that working hard in school is likely to win the support of parents and teachers, so they'll understand that appearance is just as important. And as this belief grows within them and their peers, they will start to spend more and more time assessing their own and others' appearance.

All of these factors would have had a bearing on Chloe's young life. And, around the same time she started to pay attention to her appearance, she was also starting to think differently about herself in other ways. You will have read how Chloe was a happy, active child who worked hard at school and enjoyed singing and dancing. But, following the incident when her teacher made fun of her for putting her hand up, Chloe started to become a little bit more introverted as she started worrying more about what people thought of her, causing her to retreat into herself. It started slowly at first, but her worries started to grow as she moved into secondary school, and she became more and more introverted.

From a psychological point of view, the problem wasn't just that Chloe started becoming more reserved, but it was also her belief that she had to change who she was to fit in. Of course, wanting to fit in to your social group is a very normal thing, especially for young people – this is the age when self-identity is forming. We want to have the approval of others, and we want to be accepted for who we are. Chloe felt that if she remained the same, she would be rejected in some way. Her teacher's rebuke effectively taught her to act less like herself in order to get through school successfully. She learnt that in order to feel okay at school, she needed to be the same as everyone else. Clearly that was not a very healthy lesson to have forced on her at such an impressionable age.

## IDENTIFYING THE PROBLEM

By this stage in her journey, Chloe says she felt that her life felt "wrong". This is a common evaluation for people with body image concerns; something is just not right, but you don't know what. Identifying what the actual problem is can often take time, and as with Chloe, there isn't just one single factor that contributes to how you feel, so understanding what is actually wrong can be confusing and overwhelming.

One of the reasons why so many mental health conditions go untreated for so long is that when you're growing up it can be hard to determine what is considered normal. It can be difficult to figure out what are regarded as acceptable or unacceptable feelings and behaviour.

## SELF-CRITICISM

As a consequence of believing she was different from everybody else her age, Chloe's inner critic had free rein. Self-criticism and feelings of shame aren't necessarily part and parcel of all conditions – but self-criticism and shame tend to feature strongly in cases of body dissatisfaction.

Quite often, the self-criticism can predate body dissatisfaction. The voice that one hears when suffering from body dissatisfaction is relentlessly critical, although it might not feel like that at first.

Initially, the voice might seem like a protective one – one that is only trying to safeguard you against getting humiliated or rejected. Then, as time goes on, it will start to feel like an over-zealous presence so that, instead of seeming to protect you in moments of threat, it starts trying to pre-empt situations and warn you in situations that aren't threatening at all. It all feels a bit like having a parrot on your shoulder reminding you how terrible you are, all the time.

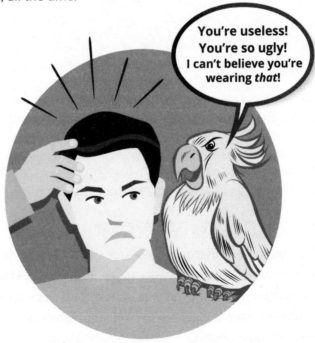

We know of course that if you continue to tell someone how useless they are, they start to believe it and behave like it is actually true.

So, Chloe's intense self-criticism is common, especially in cases where body dissatisfaction and depression are working wave by wave. Essentially it is another form of negative thinking – a form of critical self-evaluation – and we discuss this further in Part II.

## APPEARANCE IS EVERYTHING

People with body image problems and BDD place too much value on appearance, often to the exclusion of other aspects of themselves. Understandably, we live in a society that bombards us with images of "perfect" people and it is very hard to stop paying attention to these ideal images. So one of the important things we need to do is to address this disparity and restore a broader, more balanced identity and sense of self. In many cases, people need to reconnect with who they are underneath their BDD and body image concerns.

As body dissatisfaction takes hold, it is very easy for people to just view themselves in terms of their appearance and nothing else; this is the only currency that matters. They forget that they're also creative, or funny, or kind, or interesting, or interested, or passionate, or curious, or that they have many other unique qualities. They have lost the detail and the nuance of their own lives and personality, so that every little thing is seen in terms of how they look, relative to other people.

## LOSS OF PERSPECTIVE

Living with body dissatisfaction and BDD really is an all-consuming job. If somebody asks somebody who is suffering with body dissatisfaction to do something, they're immediately trying to solve the problem of how they can navigate their way through the obstacles facing them in terms of their appearance. That might be as simple as thinking *How am I going to get from A to B, without being seen?*

Let's assume someone invited Chloe out for coffee. Her first thought wouldn't have been, *Great, that'll be nice.* It would have been a succession of anxious thoughts: *How on earth am I going to get to that coffee shop? What will I be able to wear? If I get there and I need to leave, what can I say? Will I be able to get in without seeing myself in the mirror in that café? Will I be able to sit with my back to it? And how do I do all of that without my friend noticing? Maybe I should just cancel?*

Eventually there's no other dialogue in their head, other than in relation to their appearance and managing the obstacles they perceive around their appearance. They have to work really hard at it. Chloe worked incredibly hard at it. Her life was consumed by the effort.

## SAFETY BEHAVIOURS

One of the key things in tackling any body image problems or BDD is identifying and changing the unhelpful coping strategies or, as we call them, safety behaviours. These are the things that people do to reduce the chance of their perceived flaw(s) being seen, or to protect other people from having to see the perceived flaw(s). In essence, people undertake these safety behaviours to avoid or minimise what they perceive as threatening situations, and the safety behaviour offers relief from the severe anxiety they would feel if they'd had to endure the situation.

For example, if you have a concern about the size or shape of your ears, you might wear large glasses to distract people from looking at your ears. That's a safety behaviour. Another safety behaviour would be to always wear your hair down so that you cover your ears.

Typical safety behaviours by people with body image concerns and BDD include:

- Avoidance of any situations (e.g. classes, parties, and public transport), people, or things (e.g. lights, certain types of clothes, and mirrors or reflective surfaces) that might trigger anxiety over appearance
- Excessive time spent getting ready to leave the house
- Excessive checking of your appearance in the mirror or other reflective surfaces
- Camouflaging or hiding the area of concern with heavy make-up, hairstyles, or clothes
- Standing in certain positions so the area of concern is not noticed
- Dieting
- Excessive exercise
- Dermatological procedures
- Seeking cosmetic surgery
- Going to the hairdressers or beautician excessively

Please note, this is not an exhaustive list! It is just to give you a general idea of some of the more common safety behaviours. The types of safety behaviours people engage in are extremely varied and creative so there is no way we could list them all.

> **The problem with safety behaviours is that they keep the problem going, and usually make it worse**

When you carry out a safety behaviour it gives more strength to the idea that if you don't do it, people will notice the area that is giving you concern. For example, if you're used to walking around wearing a lot of make-up, you might think, *Thank goodness I'm wearing my make-up, or else people would see what I truly look like!* Thus it is reinforcing the idea that you are ugly and need to wear make-up to hide this fact from people.

So, while safety behaviours give you a sense of relief and make you feel safe from the threat of someone noticing your perceived flaw(s), these behaviours actually reinforce the worry. They won't help you change unhelpful and untrue beliefs about your appearance! We call this a vicious cycle – where the things you do to rescue yourself from the threat give the problem more power and keep it going.

## AVOIDANCE

Rather than subject themselves to certain trigger events or situations, people may use avoidance techniques. For example, in Chloe's case, she avoided wearing low-cut tops in the summer, so that her neck was not on display. Her ultimate avoidance technique was not going out at all.

## COMPULSIONS / REPETITIVE BEHAVIOURS

Compulsions, also known as repetitive behaviours, are actions that people feel compelled to engage in to try to stop a threat or obsession, e.g. people noticing the features they worry about, or thinking they're ugly. While they're more likely to apply to people suffering from BDD, actually anyone with body image problems can experience compulsions. A compulsion is a safety behaviour and is usually repeated excessively. Some common repetitive behaviours people might engage in include skin picking, mirror checking and touching their face to see how their skin feels. Compulsions can also be mental acts – things people do in their head – such as comparing themselves with others. When Chloe went out, she felt compelled to check her appearance as often as she could.

## REASSURANCE SEEKING

Reassurance seeking refers to the act of seeking reassurance from others that the body feature you worry about is not noticeable, and that you are presentable enough to be seen in public. As you'll go on to read in Chloe's story, she often resorted to reassurance seeking, particularly asking her mum if she looked okay.

Reassurance seeking is very common in body image problems and BDD. Some examples might be:

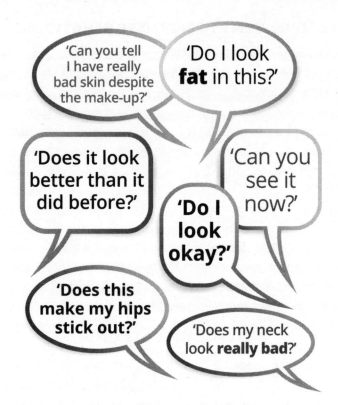

Reassurance seeking rarely, if ever, provides relief – or not the specific kind of relief that people are seeking. Even if they get a positive response, e.g. 'You look great' or 'You can't notice it', (which is what they want), they don't feel any relief because their own doubts are so entrenched. And then they will find ways to reason this reassurance away too: *They're just saying that to be nice, They don't want to hurt my feelings*, etc. There is no relief (or only very fleeting relief) because they are so convinced about how awful they look that they rarely trust what anyone says – and then the worry cycle starts again.

## UNINTENDED CONSEQUENCES

Another issue with safety behaviours is that they can actually lead to unintended consequences that might make the problem worse. For example, if you wear a hat to hide a bald spot, or you wear dark glasses to hide bags under your eyes, you might actually draw more attention to yourself, particularly if people aren't used to seeing you wear a hat or sunglasses. So the irony is that the very thing you do to try to keep attention away from yourself can in fact invite more attention!

Another example would be if you're worried about slight acne on your face and wear very heavy make-up most of the time. You might actually make the acne worse, or even cause more acne to develop. Again, the intention is to hide what you see as a problem, but the methods you use make the problem worse.

## RUMINATION

People with BDD and body image issues spend so much time in their heads assessing, reviewing, and churning over their thoughts about things that have happened – and we call this ruminating. When people ruminate, they devote intense scrutiny to past events which they replay over and over in their heads. Although it doesn't technically count as ruminating (as ruminating specifically references worrying about the past), people may also spend a great deal of time worrying about future issues. The problem with excessive ruminating and worrying about future events is that it takes the person out of the present moment. Another problem is that it doesn't provide any answers or comfort.

Actually, we all ruminate from time to time. For example, it's natural to want to replay a conversation in our heads if we feel it went particularly badly – we may believe that it can help us learn from a bad experience. But ruminating is not helpful; it is a passive process, not an active problem-solving process. It pushes all your other mental processes into the background, but doesn't offer you any solutions. People who ruminate habitually often find that hours pass without them really even knowing what they've been doing. It is a cyclical train of thought that can quickly become obsessive.

After her grandmother died, Chloe was aware that she was becoming more and more internalised. Instead of talking about her feelings, she was bottling up her experiences and worries and dwelling on them. She dwelled upon her guilt about the circumstances surrounding her grandmother's stroke, and ruminated on what she could have done differently. She ruminated on her morbid thoughts. And part of the issue with Chloe ruminating is that she just had too much time to think. It's very easy to ruminate when you're not interacting with another person who commands your attention.

The key to addressing rumination is learning to identify when you are doing it, and then being able to shift your focus away from your thoughts and on to something else. We address ways to stop ruminating in Part II.

## SELECTIVE ATTENTION

Selective attention or hyper-vigilance is when you focus on information that you perceive as a threat, and use that information to reinforce unhelpful beliefs. It is found in all BDD and body image problems. We can see that selective attention might seem like a positive way to focus on information. For example, if you are driving on a foggy night and you have to follow the cat's eyes lights and the road lines very carefully, it makes sense to pay attention to those things to the exclusion of other distractions, so that you make it home safely. But in body image problems and BDD, selective attention can be counterproductive. For example, if Chloe was in town, she would scan everyone's reactions to see if they were looking at her and noticing how ugly she was. Inevitably, because she was scanning everyone, she would notice it just as soon as someone glanced at her, even momentarily, and then interpret it as evidence that she was grotesque. However, if you are going about your day-to-day business without scanning other people's reactions, then you wouldn't even notice if someone did glance at you.

Here's an experiment that helps demonstrate selective attention:

> Take 30 seconds and stare at your little finger. Try to notice every tiny, little detail.
>
> Once the time is up, what did you notice? Did you notice more detail the longer you looked?

Now, if you ask somebody else to describe your little finger, they won't be able to tell you very much at all. You have been intently focused on it. You have selectively focused on your finger without distraction, so you're aware of every little mark, whereas the other person won't have given it a moment's thought.

So the problem now is that, when you selectively attend to things to the exclusion of anything else, you become more convinced about how unmissable your "problem" is. This reinforces the safety behaviours in which you are engaging.

## SELF-FOCUSED ATTENTION

People suffering with body image issues and BDD often get caught up in self-focused attention. Self-focused attention is like being lost in your own head. It happens when an individual focuses all their attention on how they're feeling or how they're going to be perceived. For example, you may be in conversation with someone, but you're so overwhelmed with feeling anxious that you only pay attention to anxiety. Then you start to wonder if the other person can tell how anxious you are. You are no longer paying full attention to the conversation.

Focusing in on yourself like this means that there isn't any room for other information to give you a wider perspective on the situation. When you are in the situation that we described above, you think your face is red or your cheeks are flushed and the other person is looking at you because they can see these visible signs, making you even more self-conscious. This all feeds back into your anxiety and encourages you to go on monitoring yourself.

## PERFECTIONISM

Perfectionism refers to striving compulsively for impossible goals. People may also set excessively high standards for their performance. This means they will be very self-critical when they don't hit these targets. They may strive for perfection in one or more areas of their life.

Obviously, people with body image issues and BDD will be more focused on their appearance and set incredibly high standards for themselves, which will be impossible for them to live up to. People with body image problems and BDD who experience perfectionism not only become very self-critical, but also may end up avoiding things such as going out and socialising because getting ready involves so much effort to achieve their desired standard of appearance.

# CHAPTER 3

# BAD THERAPY

 ***Chloe:*** It was summer 2010, I was 17 years old, and I'd spent the best part of the year at home – most of it in bed.

Mum asked me again if I'd like to do my A Levels. I didn't know if I would be able to manage it, but I didn't want to disappoint her. I knew how much she was worrying about me. And I knew I had to try to do *something*.

She managed to find me a little tutorial college in Brighton for one-to-one tuition. I was still wary of the idea of going back into education, but I took a look around and met the course supervisor. She already knew all about me – Mum had thought it best to tell her everything – and she was really encouraging.

On the one hand, I was apprehensive about having to commute so far to college, but on the other hand, it didn't feel like a normal school. I'd always really hated the thought of getting into trouble with teachers at school (if I'd been absent at any point, I'd always made sure I got a sick note from Mum). But here, everything was designed to be a lot more flexible. I knew that I wouldn't have to go in if I didn't feel up to it – and I wouldn't get into trouble for it.

So I decided to do it. Getting the train every day was an ordeal in itself. But I was desperate to make it work. While my sister and my old friends were moving on with their lives, I was in limbo, and I was desperate to catch up.

I chose law, psychology, and film. I was getting more and more passionate about film and, in particular, film criticism, so the idea of being able to study film was a real inspiration. I liked all of my teachers, and my course supervisor was a wonderful source of support – she was a very empathetic human being.

Between September and November, I managed to keep up a fairly regular attendance. But after that, it dropped quickly. The journey was very, very hard. I hated being seen by so many people. I knew that every one of them was judging my appearance and seeing all my flaws.

I knew Mum would be devastated. We had never really talked about what I was going through, not properly. Every time we'd tried to discuss it, it had felt like I was stuttering through the words and that everything was coming out wrong. But I needed her to know that I was hurting inside. So I wrote her a letter to try to articulate how I was feeling:

*I don't really know how to start this letter. All I know is that I need help. I'm frightened for my future and I don't know what to do. I can't take it any more. I'm sick of being the person left behind with nothing to show. Is it too late? Is all my motivation gone?*

*I feel like I've let everyone down, like I'm the family secret. I want to get on with my life because I feel like I've wasted my youth. I know I won't be the person I once was, but I've got to find a way to cope.*

*I guess in a way this is my final cry for help.*

That was the catalyst. After Mum read it, she said we had to see a doctor. And this time I knew I couldn't say no.

My doctor decided I was depressed. He started me on 20mg of fluoxetine, a Selective Serotonin Reuptake Inhibitor (SSRI), in December and put me on a waiting list for a course of Cognitive Behavioural Therapy (CBT). The antidepressant helped ... but only for a little while.

At the same time, I was having driving lessons and although they were going okay, I found the gears quite difficult, and the stress of it was really getting to me. My sister had already passed her theory test, but I couldn't face the prospect of failing, so I quit instead of risking it. I said that I wanted to focus on my A Levels instead, but deep down, I knew I was just saying that to make myself believe it.

A year after starting my A Levels, I was really struggling with my attendance. I still went to see my film teacher and my psychology teacher when I felt like I was able to. Everyone was incredibly understanding, but I suppose that just made it even easier for me to decide not to go. I knew I wouldn't get into trouble for not going, so it made it easier to justify staying at home if I felt insecure. And my insecurity was all-encompassing now. When I look back and see everything that I was missing out on, I realised what a compromised life I was living. People my age were having fun, while I was hiding – not going out, not socialising, just staying in my room. I hated myself. I hated my appearance. And I knew my life was over. I didn't live. I just existed. As the stress began to take its toll, I knew I needed a release, a way out. And then I found one ...

Whenever I felt really frustrated or annoyed with myself, I would cut myself. Whenever I tried to motivate myself to do something positive, and then failed, I would cut myself. It wasn't a regular thing, but I needed to know it was there for me if I needed it – the only way I knew to stop ruminating on all the negative thoughts that were crashing in on me.

Self-harm became a way out. I quickly got locked into a cycle of punishing myself for not being good enough. I would get so angry, but I didn't have any other way to express how I felt. It was the classic thing of trying to show how you feel on the inside – on the outside. A strange mix of punishment and relief.

I'd just take scissors or whatever was lying around, and do it on my forearm, or the tops of my thighs. I never did it too deep – I didn't want to go to hospital, it wasn't an attempt to end my life. It wasn't even a cry for help; everyone already knew I was in pain. So it was more about getting some temporary relief. It just had to be enough for me to get some relief from the emotional pain. Physical pain gave me something else to focus on. And I made sure I looked as I did it; it hurt more when I could see myself doing it.

It was so hard to express my feelings, even with my family. I remember when my dad bought Mother's Day lunch, and I really didn't want to go, so I left getting ready until the last minute. Mum told me how much it would mean to her if I was there and Olivia told me to just do it for Mum. So I tried. I really tried. I washed, but didn't put any make-up on. Then I just broke down in the lounge.

I couldn't take the guilt I felt and I didn't know how to express all my emotions, disappointment, and shame. I'd had years of feeling like the rubbish child, and I couldn't take any more. I knew they couldn't understand, but I tried to tell them. I said that mentally and physically I just couldn't go. I was shaking so hard – it was almost like a physical outpouring. I think it was a build-up of all the times I hadn't felt able to go out before, but hadn't been able to say no. I don't think I had ever come to terms with just how draining my life had become.

That sort of extreme reaction was a one-off. I had learnt to be a lot more reserved: a lot more British! Usually the only way I could express my feelings was on my own, in my room, when everyone else was asleep. That was when the tears came and I broke down, all alone. Or else I'd focus in on the pain and cut myself some more.

There'd been times when I'd gone to Mum at night, but I'd never been able to really open up to her. Not like that. She knew it was difficult. She knew that if she encouraged me it usually helped, but there were times when it did the opposite.

I still had a few friends – and some of them still tried to reach out to me. From their perspective, the idea of us getting together for lunch would seem like nothing. But to me, it was a huge commitment. I could only imagine the worst possible outcomes, and I hardly ever managed to go. After making my excuses, I'd ruminate about the whole thing. I'd play it through in my mind and wonder if it would've been better to have had the experience that I'd now missed out on. The missed opportunities were piling up, and more and more potential memories were passing me by.

Even to this day, there are times when I just can't do things, when my BDD rears up or depression pulls me under. I'm lucky that my family understands me so much better now. But it still gets to me. Every time I let someone down, it hurts.

I have spent so much of my life feeling guilty that I've disappointed my family and let so many people down. I especially hated disappointing my mum that Mother's Day. After everything she'd done and everything she'd endured for me, I still couldn't do that one simple thing for her in return. I felt like the worst human being ever.

There were times when I wondered about what sort of person I could have been. What would I have been like if I wasn't so withdrawn? I didn't even know what was happening to me, but I couldn't help thinking that, if I had been "normal," I could have been this great child – someone for my parents and my grandparents to be truly proud of.

It was infuriating. But it didn't matter how much I raged against it, I couldn't operate like other people my age. Sometimes I felt that I wasn't trying hard enough, but then I also felt that if I tried hard and still couldn't do it, I would feel like an even bigger failure.

And so I kept self-harming. There was a lot of information about it on Tumblr, the blogging and social networking site. There were people on there boasting about doing it – almost as if there was a certain cachet to it – and there were even tips on what to do and how to do it. It didn't feel self-destructive to me. I had no sense of self to preserve, and I had no future. I'd lost my grandparents, and I was a burden on my family. I knew I wasn't going to get better.

It was my own form of release. Just a temporary escape – something else to think about other than the usual negative spiral of destructive thoughts. I didn't want to upset my family any more and I certainly didn't want to add anything else to their list of worries about me. But I remember when my mum found out. I'd taken a shower and was leaving the bathroom with a towel on when she saw the scars. Of course she was upset. But I couldn't explain it to her. I couldn't put into words how it helped me. How can you explain something like that to the people you love when you see the pain and the sadness in their eyes? Olivia would plead with me to just open up and tell her what was wrong, but it just wasn't that easy. It never had been. After that, they were all hyper-vigilant around me and of course that annoyed me even more. I was worried they were going to hide all the knives and I hated the embarrassment I caused.

The cuts were never really deep – I was too scared for that – and they didn't need stitches. But I didn't let the wounds heal. So if I was upset or anxious, I'd rub the scars to make them hurt, or I'd try to re-open the cuts. I knew my triggers and I could recognise the wave of negative emotions building up until I had to hurt myself again.

I don't think I could have harmed myself to the point where I put my life in danger, but if it had happened accidentally, or if I had been hit by a car, then I don't think it would have upset me. I just wanted to switch my brain off. The negative voice just went on getting louder and louder, until it was the only voice in the room. And then, when the self-harm wasn't enough, I started to research ways of killing myself. I never thought I'd really be able to go through with it though. I couldn't stop thinking about what would happen if it went wrong.

In the end, I suppose I stopped because it wasn't private any more. I was doing it to help myself, but I knew it was hurting my family. So, apart from a couple of occasions later, I stopped for them. I couldn't stand the thought that they were looking at me wondering if I was self-harming.

Eventually, I learnt to replace self-harm with songs that made me sad. The songs were short enough to pay attention to, while being familiar enough that I didn't have to concentrate on them too much. I knew the songs and how they made me feel. I didn't have the right professional support structure at that stage, so I had to find my own way and I found that the right song was just able to release something.

But of course, it wasn't nearly enough. I was still trying to treat the symptoms of my condition, and I wasn't anywhere near to finding a cure. The fluoxetine wasn't doing anything for me and we were still waiting for a CBT referral. Mum decided things were so bad that we decided to seek help privately.

It was time to challenge my preconceptions. I didn't know it yet, but this was going to be the lowest part of my journey towards recovery.

Mum found a private practitioner and I went for three sessions of Cognitive Behavioural Therapy that used exposure therapy. Body dysmorphia wasn't mentioned to me at that point.

I found out that exposure therapy was a part of CBT that can help you face the thing that's causing your distress. It's used a lot to help people overcome phobias and other anxiety problems.

Later, I learnt just how effective exposure therapy can be in combating BDD. But I know that there is also a very fine balance between being ready for exposure therapy and being pushed into it. On this occasion, I was pushed, headlong. But, because she was a professional (and because I have never been very good at saying no to people in case I upset them), I didn't feel like I could say that I didn't feel ready. The therapist was adamant: 'You're doing it!' And so, without any preparation, we went out onto the street to begin my exposure therapy and see if people really were looking at me and judging me.

So, we went out into this little village. She told me to look directly at someone as we walked past. It was only a very small place and the pavements weren't even particularly big, so it felt unnatural. I didn't know if she wanted it to feel like that, but it made me feel horribly uncomfortable. Normally you might glance at someone as you pass, but you just see a snapshot of that person and then move on. But this was different.

An older man was walking towards us, and the therapist told me to look at him and see what he did. She wanted me to try to gauge his reaction. I didn't think that I could do it. I was worried that a) he was going to see how ugly I was and b) he was going to think I was weird.

We carried on up the road towards this man. My heart was racing. I was shaking with nerves. I didn't understand what I was doing. If this was what therapy was all about, I didn't want it. And it felt so wrong that Mum was paying all that money for me to feel so horrendous. It was absolutely excruciating. Therapy was pointless. Why did anyone bother with it? And yet, in spite of myself, I looked. And of course, it was so obvious that I was staring in a really unnatural way. So he looked back, and he must have wondered why I was staring at him.

I pulled my eyes away and felt a surge of relief. I'd done it. I'd got through it. But then the therapist made me pick another person, and then another. I knew I couldn't do it again though. It was just too excruciating. So I had to pretend I was looking, but I quickly moved my eyes away, so I couldn't really see them properly. It was the only way I could get through it. Afterwards, I couldn't be honest with her about what had happened. I just wanted to get away as fast as I could.

The therapist hadn't prepared me for the exposure. She hadn't talked me through the process or given it any kind of intellectual context. She had just made me stare at people indiscriminately. There was no learning involved whatsoever. And it was humiliating. For someone with BDD, it was about as unpleasant an experience as you can imagine. I never wanted to try therapy ever again. I genuinely didn't want to go back. It had been completely counter productive.

I felt utterly hopeless at that point. All my research had told me that exposure therapy would be the answer, but it wasn't. I didn't know what else was left. At that time, I didn't think I could try again with a different therapist. As far as I was concerned, I was out of options. In my mind, I started playing out all the worst possible outcomes of life now. I didn't know where else to turn.

That one experience could have written off therapy for me for ever. It could have ended my recovery in an instant.

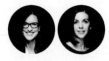 **_Lauren and Annemarie:_** Before she came to see us, Chloe had tried generic counselling and it hadn't helped. There is a difference between a generic approach to counselling and evidence-based therapy. Evidence-based treatments have been tested in laboratory settings and are scientifically proven to work. While generic counselling can be useful in a supportive way, it doesn't necessarily equip you with the tools needed to understand and change the problem, and most importantly it hasn't been proven to treat the problem.

As you'll see in Part II, this book uses evidence-based treatment protocols, based on proven techniques for addressing the unhelpful thinking patterns, emotional distress and maladaptive behaviours associated with body image problems and BDD. These include Exposure and Response Prevention (ERP), which Chloe mentioned, and this is a way of facing our fears without engaging in the safety behaviours or avoidance that you are currently caught up in. So, you can use this book as your template for addressing your body image issues and BDD.

Following the generic counselling, Chloe had a few sessions of CBT with exposure therapy. After her first experience of exposure therapy, she thought it was all over, that she'd had her one shot at BDD-specific therapy and it hadn't worked. Fortunately, it is not a one-time-only offer. Indeed, it is very common for people who have a less than successful experience of therapy to think they are untreatable, but that is not the case. There are lots of reasons why therapy might not be successful. Here are just a few of them:

- The complexity of many conditions means that they cannot be addressed and resolved using one kind of treatment. Sometimes subtler variations in treatment might be required.

- The therapist may not have understood the problem properly, or there was no shared understanding of the problem.

- There was not a good patient–therapist relationship (which may be for lots of reasons).

- Perhaps the person having treatment just wasn't ready to engage in some of the strategies, or depression or another life stressor clouded the issue and made it difficult to undertake the treatment.

If you are in the situation that you have tried therapy that hasn't worked, don't blame yourself. As you can see, there are many reasons why therapy may not be successful, or is only marginally effective. It may have been the wrong time, or the wrong therapist, or even the wrong type of treatment.

We encourage you to keep going: work through this book and, if needed, seek out another appropriately trained therapist. In fact, when seeing a therapist, we would encourage you to ask about their qualifications and whether they have treated body image problems before. Therapists have different specialty areas and use different approaches in treatment, so it is helpful to find out what type of treatment your therapist uses, and whether they have treated these problems before. You wouldn't go to a dentist to have knee surgery!

A good course of individually tailored Cognitive Behavioural Therapy is a good first step in addressing body image issues and BDD. The treatment should help you build an individualised model of your own problem, challenge unhelpful thoughts and beliefs, tolerate the difficult emotions, and change the unhelpful (or maladaptive) behaviours. And this also provides us with a structured approach to treatment.

## ENTRENCHED BELIEFS

As we have mentioned, unhelpful beliefs about ourselves and our appearance can get entrenched (or stuck). To give you an example of how beliefs might become stuck, here's an example from Annemarie's life:

*Annemarie:* After travelling for a bit, I was the first person to move into a house-share property on a street with a slightly bad reputation. I opened the door, threw all my stuff in, and chose my bedroom. While I was upstairs, the doorbell rang, but by the time I'd got downstairs and clambered over all my stuff in the hall, there was no one there when I opened the door. That's the reality, that's fact. But I then had to make sense of what I had just encountered. (And this is how beliefs are developed.) So I developed an idea that somebody had rung the wrong door, realised their mistake, and – because I'd taken a while to get there – just gone away. Or, they had rung the right door, but because I'd taken too long to get to the door, they'd just moved on. And that was all fine. It made sense to me and I just forgot about it and carried on.

A couple of days later, the bell rang – and this time it was quite late at night. So I went downstairs, and because I was feeling slightly cautious, I wasn't in any great hurry to get to the door. I'd only let a couple of people know that I'd moved in, so I was wondering who would be ringing at this time of night. I opened the door and there was nobody there.

So now I'd discounted my first idea because that didn't fit with what I was experiencing any more, and I'd moved on to an alternative interpretation of events. So then I thought it was probably kids messing about. I thought they must have rung the bell and run away, so I closed the door and just tried to ignore it.

A few days later, it happened again. But this time, it was three o'clock in the morning! I looked out of the bay window to try to see down by the front door. But I just couldn't make anything out. I certainly didn't want to open the door, and I was scared now. I'd discounted my first two theories and moved onto a third theory – and that's when I decided that someone was playing some nasty tricks on me. The bell ringing went on for the best part of two weeks, and at the end of that time, I had convinced myself that I didn't want to stay there any more. I had started to look out of the window and see unsavoury characters hanging around outside the house. I was developing new beliefs about the people I was seeing, and about myself as well. I had just come back from four months travelling around the world independently, and now I saw myself as vulnerable. So I went from feeling very assured and capable to feeling unsure about myself, and that the world was more dangerous than I had previously thought.

Then on a Saturday morning, a letter dropped through the door. It was from my landlady, and it said the doorbell was faulty! But no worries, the letter reassured me, because she'd come over and fitted a new battery so I shouldn't have any more problems with it. That possibility had never even occurred to me. But now, if something like that were to happen again, it would be one of my first theories.

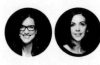 ***Lauren and Annemarie:*** As you can see from Annemarie's story, there can be alternative explanations of events, but you are unlikely to consider them if you are filtering the information to support an already predetermined idea. The "unsavoury" characters Annemarie noticed were probably just going out, or waiting to meet somebody. But because Annemarie was interpreting the situation as a threat, she experienced this as yet another piece of

evidence that she was right – that her neighbourhood was dangerous. That is how belief systems work.

Let's say Annemarie hadn't received the letter from the landlady and had left that property and moved elsewhere. She would have still held the belief that she was vulnerable, and would have chosen places to live in a different way – maybe favouring "safer" neighbourhoods, or properties with different security features etc.

The reality is that in therapy, we would identify that the belief exists, identify when it began, how it developed, and what maintains it. In this example, one of the things Annemarie did to maintain the belief that she lived in a dangerous neighbourhood was making sure she wasn't in the house on her own. But even if the neighbourhood was not dangerous, and it was just a faulty doorbell, she was living like it was a dangerous place and that made her feel scared and vulnerable.

So, in our treatment programme we try to change the stuck entrenched beliefs, because they have either developed subjectively, or are probably not based on reality.

## TAKING A DIFFERENT PERSPECTIVE

One of Chloe's typical beliefs would be that she if she walked down the street, people would think that she was repulsive and she would feel humiliated. Then, as a result of her humiliation, the rest of her day would be ruined and she would hide indoors. But that becomes a self-fulfilling prophecy,[5] because her fear of potential humiliation means that she stays inside and her day is ruined anyway.

Chloe didn't have any other possible interpretations. She said they were staring because she was ugly, whereas there might have been a number of other reasons people were looking at her. But it was just difficult for Chloe to think of them at the time. With some encouragement, she was able to generate some other reasons why they might have been looking:

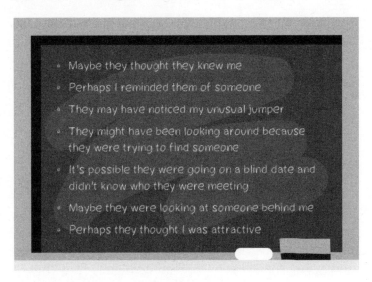

- Maybe they thought they knew me
- Perhaps I reminded them of someone
- They may have noticed my unusual jumper
- They might have been looking around because they were trying to find someone
- It's possible they were going on a blind date and didn't know who they were meeting
- Maybe they were looking at someone behind me
- Perhaps they thought I was attractive

Even if some of the alternate reasons may feel hard to believe, we still add them to the list because we're coming up with all sorts of possibilities, regardless of how likely you think they are. You might say your original interpretation feels like the right one, but there are actually several plausible explanations.

Our beliefs about things can feel very real, even if we don't have the evidence to back them up. But evidence-based therapy doesn't say that your belief or interpretation is wrong; it just requires you to accept that there are other possible interpretations and asks you to try to see things from other perspectives. So it's not about putting on rose-tinted glasses and pretending the original interpretation is not true, but it does provide the possibility that there are other, potentially more realistic and less threatening explanations.

Very often, there is no one right answer. Life isn't that straightforward. We're almost always going to have alternatives. So, we just pick the one that seems the most plausible. As we've mentioned, the purpose of CBT is not to falsely create positive thinking. It is to encourage helpful and more realistic thinking – for example, conceding that the way you interpret the situation isn't the only way. In the example where someone appeared to stare at Chloe, her initial thought that they were starting at her because she was ugly might well be correct. But we're just asking her to accept that, although she might not feel like the alternatives are true, they might be. And in fact, as it turns out, her alternative ideas provide many more likely explanations.

If we do then assume one of the alternative explanations are true, what difference would that make to how Chloe lived and what she did? It might mean that she would:

- Feel less anxious, and be more likely to go out again
- Stop interpreting other people looking at her as a threatening situation
- Not feel the need to hide or disguise her neck and other features
- Spend less time getting ready to go out

And most importantly, each time she did one of these things and realised that she wasn't being stared at or she wasn't being told she was ugly, she would start to build evidence for her – more helpful – alternative belief.

## SELF-HARM

Chloe talked about how she started self-harming in response to the emotional pain that she was experiencing. Although it is often misunderstood, self-harm is usually a way of trying to distract from difficult feelings, or to show other people you are hurting emotionally. People can self-harm in a number of ways, but the most common is cutting. And it is important to note that people who self-harm are not always intending to kill themselves. So if you are reading this in concern because you have found out that somebody you love or care about is self-harming, that does not always mean that they are likely to try to kill themselves. Indeed, as Chloe explained, she was careful to avoid causing any serious, lasting damage. However, it can be the case that sometimes when people self-harm, the injuries can become infected, or they may accidentally injure themselves severely and require medical attention immediately. Therefore, we still consider self-harm a serious health issue. So if you are self-harming, or you know someone who is, we recommend that you speak with a health professional who can help you find some better coping methods. Also, please read Part II Section 1, where we show you how to deal with distressing emotions and find alternative ways to manage these feelings, without having to resort to self-harming.

# CHAPTER 4

## GIVING MY ILLNESS A NAME

**Chloe:** At the start of 2012, aged 18, I was seen by my local child mental health team. We talked over my case history and discussed it with the multi-disciplinary team. We talked about my grandparents and my friends at school, but we didn't get to the root of anything. It was just a Band-Aid.

I wasn't sleeping well and that was affecting my desire and ability to go to college. They put me on mirtazapine, a tetracyclic antidepressant, and referred me to the Time to Talk (TTT) service. After an initial assessment with the TTT team, they put me on a four-month waiting list. During that time, I saw the nurse fairly regularly, and I liked her. I felt like I'd seen a lot of people who hadn't really tried to empathise with me, so it made a big difference. I opened up to her a little bit more than with others.

The mirtazapine helped me to sleep, but it had a side effect – carbohydrate craving – and I put on about two stone (12.5 kg) in weight in a very short time. There were purply red stretch marks radiating out past my belly button, and I felt horrible.

I'd always been a healthy weight, if not very slim. Sometimes I had put on a bit of extra weight here and there, but nothing too bad. Nothing that really affected my confidence. But that extra weight from taking the medication really sent my body image problem into overdrive.

I saw the mental health nurse in May and told her how unhappy I was about the carbohydrate craving, and how it was affecting my confidence. She arranged for me to see a psychiatrist, who took me off the mirtazapine and increased my dosage of fluoxetine to 40mg. By the time he saw me again two weeks later, the mirtazapine had worn off and the sleeplessness had returned. But he thought it would settle and said he wouldn't be able to see me again because he was leaving the hospital.

I still wasn't sleeping, but as far as he was concerned, it would settle down in time. And that was that! There was nothing more he could do for me. I was on my own again. There was no plan. No way forward. No reassurance.

Without sleep and without motivation I couldn't face going back to college. The prospect of taking (and potentially failing) exams was terrifying. I had promised Mum I would, but when it came to it, I just wasn't ready. In my head, I had already convinced myself I couldn't pass – and I certainly couldn't have risked it because failing the exams would only have added to my feelings of not being good enough. I wrote Mum another letter to tell her how I was feeling; it was easier than talking about my feelings, but it was only really scratching the surface.

It was time to be open, or at least as open as I could be. She needed to know that it wasn't an occasional issue; that I was constantly worried about people looking at me and what they would think of me. I told her that every day is a struggle when you can't stand the person you see in the mirror. I told her about the day I went to London with my friend, and about how self-conscious I had felt on the Tube. I explained how sure I was that every single person was looking at me, judging me, finding me repulsive. I told her how it felt when I saw a girl in a shop who, in my mind, was perfect – she was everything I wanted to be. She was buying all these expensive clothes and as I watched her, it all came crashing in on me – all the hurt, the anguish and the bleakness of my existence. I was mortified. I just wanted to run and hide in my bedroom and shut out the world so that no one would ever have to see my face again.

I told Mum I was sorry: sorry about all the money they were paying for college. Sorry for letting everyone down. But in my heart of hearts, I knew I was as low as I had ever been. I was trapped. Now that I had been discharged, I felt as if I had nowhere to go, except back to my GP. I trusted her at least. I knew she was genuinely trying to help me. But it felt like going back to square one.

I was referred to a consultant psychiatrist, and I saw him in August. He had a different take on things. He didn't think I was suffering from depression and recommended I come off the antidepressants and suggested a course of CBT. I saw the therapist a couple of times but it didn't help. I didn't particularly like his style – it was much too general, and it didn't really address my main issues. But one thing he said made perfect sense – and it was the first time it had ever been suggested. He told me he thought I was suffering from Body Dysmorphic Disorder.

I knew I was low, but even then, mental health issues weren't really on my radar. I certainly hadn't heard of BDD. Mental health was never discussed when I was at school, and I barely knew anything about it. I thought that to be mentally ill you had to be sectioned. I didn't understand the gradients and I didn't understand why my brain was making me feel this way. But I looked at the symptoms with Mum and thought that they described me exactly.

Just having a possible diagnosis didn't change how I felt, but it gave me a new perspective on things. To me it felt like one chapter was ending and another one was starting. There was a sense of relief, I suppose. I wasn't the only one. I wasn't acting out, or being strange. *The piece of the puzzle fits*, I thought.

My mum was glad to have an answer. My dad found it harder to understand – but it is difficult to understand. The concept of body image was so alien to him. My sister was concerned, but also relieved there was an answer. When there's an answer, hopefully there's a solution.

For a long time, I had wanted to feel and look "better" than I was. But did having BDD mean I was vain? Not at all. There wasn't a hint of vanity. And I didn't think I had a skewed sense of my own self. My sense of my own identity was absolute: I was ugly. Like a gargoyle. That was all there was to it.

Looking back, I know I wasn't seeing things clearly, but at the time I had absolutely no doubt about it. I couldn't understand how people didn't see what I could see. I thought they were just being nice when they protested.

I said "gargoyle." It's such a brutal way to describe someone. But it fits, because what you see is so disfigured and distorted. It's almost like you're somehow removed from reality and looking at yourself from a different perspective, like an out-of-body experience. Or a nightmare.

For me, there wasn't a sudden onset of BDD. It wasn't like I woke up one morning and thought I was ugly. For me, it was quite a gradual process and it snowballed from there. It happened in little increments. So, for example, I would notice something on my face, and to begin with I might have only noticed it once a week. But then gradually it became once a day, then once an hour. My reality became warped bit by bit.

It doesn't take much to change your reality. I remember a girl at school who said I was ugly, but I didn't have very much respect for her – and neither did many other people. She was quite loud and brash, so her opinion didn't really affect me and I was able to brush it off. But sometimes, someone can say something to you, and – even if you don't respect them – that thing can change your whole reality.

I think the roots of BDD are, partly, individual (something inside you that makes you susceptible to it) and partly environmental (the experiences you have and the things people say).

I remember when my sister mentioned my neck. I don't think I'd ever really noticed it until one day, on holiday, I was wearing a dress and she looked at me strangely and said, 'Your neck's sticking out a little bit.' She said it was because I was standing at a funny angle. And that's when I first latched on to the idea that my neck was sticking out. That's when my reality started to change some more. One day my neck was fine, and then it wasn't. After that, my paranoia grew more and more. Soon, I was checking it from every angle – which was obviously quite difficult. Eventually I resorted to covering it up with a scarf, so nobody else could see it.

So for me, there was a gradual emergence of the insecurities that had begun in school. In part, it depended on my mood – the worse my state of mind, the more warped my reality would be. And because it took so long to get a diagnosis, my reality wasn't ever challenged. There was just my belief and I was collecting evidence to back up my beliefs. The longer they went unchallenged, the worse it got. As my new reality took hold, I became increasingly overwhelmed and obsessed by my BDD.

But why hadn't I noticed something was wrong? Surely I should have known that the way I thought about myself was problematic in some way? At the time, I just thought it was part and parcel of depression and anxiety.

A lot of people with BDD seek reassurance from the people around them. I did that too. But if I ever asked Mum if I looked okay, or even if she just said something nice of her own volition, I'd just assume she was saying it because that's what mums do. Mums say nice things to make their kids feel better. I sought reassurance for the things I was already most concerned about. So I wouldn't ask, 'Do I look alright?' I would ask, 'Does my neck stick out?

Is my scarf covering everything?' But no matter what was said to reassure me, I never believed it. You only ever take on board the things that fit your ideology.

**So now I had a diagnosis of BDD. What next?**

There were no BDD services in Sussex, so we started googling. Our research came up with Professor David Veale's name – the leading specialist on BDD – who helped write the NICE clinical guidelines. (The National Institute for Health and Care Excellence provides the most up-to-date advice and guidance to help improve healthcare in the UK.) My doctor referred us and we got an appointment at the Priory in July 2013. I was a bit nervous about going because I'd heard of the Priory as the famous place where the celebrities went when they were recovering from alcoholism or drug addiction.

Professor Veale diagnosed BDD, social anxiety, and depression. He put me back on antidepressants, starting me off on 20mg of citalopram (also known as Celexa or Cipramil), another SSRI, which increased to 40mg after a couple of weeks. I wasn't confident that it was going to make any difference, but he told me that different medications had different effects on different people, so I persisted.

The things Professor Veale told me made about BDD and its wide range of potential impacts made a lot of sense to me. I felt abnormally ugly, but Professor Veale told me that was common for people suffering with BDD. I learnt that some people fixated on a specific physical feature, whereas others worried about a range of features. I fell into both camps. I worried about skin tone, facial hair, and body hair, but my neck had become my biggest source of concern. I was conscious of the way it protruded – almost as if the top of my neck wasn't straight.

So Professor Veale asked me to draw a picture of my face and neck, so I could show him what I thought I looked like. I was quite embarrassed – I thought he was going to judge me on my drawing – so I found it difficult. I didn't know if I could accurately draw what I saw when I looked in the mirror. But I drew it all, and afterwards, he got me to explain what each part meant.

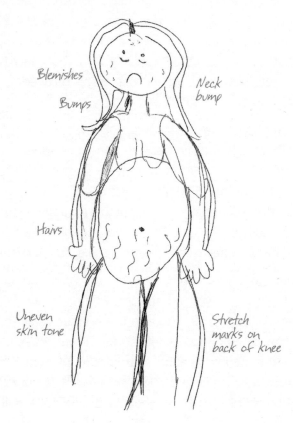

I talked him through the pores and the hair and the uneven skin tone and the eyebrows, and I told him about the hump on my neck. When I'd finished, seeing it all on paper was a bit overwhelming. I felt like crying. But he couldn't reconcile what he saw in the picture with what he saw when he looked at me. He said, 'I can't see any of those things.' And I knew that a thousand people could have said the same thing to me and it wouldn't have made a blind bit of difference. But if he couldn't see the problems, how was he supposed to help me?

Professor Veale also explained the fight, flight, or freeze response to me. He told me that when we experience anxiety, adrenaline surges through our body. This is a natural response to a highly pressured situation: it's what gave the cavemen the extra strength they needed to outrun predators or take them on in a fight. We still get that adrenaline surge today, when we are in danger. So we can choose to stand our ground and fight, or run away. In some cases we will freeze and play dead. The problem happens if we get that adrenaline surge and the threat we think we're facing isn't actually real, or it's much smaller than we imagined.

I realised that I had been locked in flight mode for most of the last three years. I would just run, physically or emotionally, from my problems, just so I could avoid confronting them.

As well as BDD, I was diagnosed with co-morbid depression and social anxiety disorder. The social anxiety disorder made me feel sick about the prospect of going out in public. And it was impossible for me to go out without thinking that everybody would be looking at me. It all added to my growing sense of alienation.

I decided to tell some people about my diagnosis. Just a few. While it was good to open up, I wondered if they'd judge me. But I had got to the point where I had to say something and explain what was happening to me. Everyone else was achieving things, even little things that were completely beyond me. I now had a diagnosis of BDD, but I was still stuck.

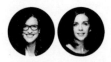 *Lauren and Annemarie:* Is there a specific trigger for body image issues and BDD? Sometimes. But equally, the emergence of body image issues and BDD can be more gradual.

Some people have a really specific memory of the onset of their body image issues and BDD. The most common trigger tends to be an emotionally charged experience, where embarrassment or shame became associated with a given body part. This experience may be a one-off, or it could be part of a collection of subsequent experiences, such as bullying. Perhaps they saw a photo of themselves and had a sudden realisation that their nose looked big, or their skin looked uneven. Perhaps someone said something to them – not necessarily something intended to hurt them. It could have just been an innocent, offhand remark. Or it could even be that they were watching TV and they saw a character and thought, *But my ears look like that!* So, there are times when it can be a realisation – a moment when it really kicks in.

But for some people, it will manifest very gradually, beginning with a low level of dissatisfaction with a given body part. Initially that may take the form of wishing their nose was smaller or that their complexion was fairer or their thighs were smaller. There aren't any physical activities associated with their emerging dissatisfaction at this point. But, over time, the person may begin to spend longer in the bathroom, working on their complexion, finding ways to arrange their hair to make their nose appear less prominent, or start dieting and exercising purely to lose weight around their thighs.

The onset often coincides with adolescence, when young people's sense of their own appearance comes into focus as a part of growing up. The repeated attention they give to their "flaws" and the negative emotional responses gradually build until what was once a relatively harmless habit or mild concern turns into a fully blown obsession, accompanied by crippling anxiety.

Body dissatisfaction may be related to obvious triggers like bullying, where the person is subjected to an influx of negative comments. But it can also result from the absence of positive comments that the person used to get. For example, if you get used to family and friends saying, 'Oh you're such a pretty girl!' and then people stop saying that to you, it's easy to notice that absence of positive feedback and focus instead on what is not being said. In this case, the easy assumption to make is that you are not praiseworthy for being pretty any more.

We believe the onset of Chloe's BDD was gradual. Chloe remembered the incident where she put her hand up in class as being especially painful. It isn't necessarily the case that everything started there, but it was probably a trigger for acute self-consciousness / awareness. Where previously she was a happy-go-lucky child who enjoyed life without reservations, she was suddenly faced with uncertainty. For the first time, Chloe began to worry about what other people might think of her, which can be a precursor for body dysmorphia.

Chloe mentioned the incident where her sister told her that her neck looked strange. But how does one remark like that come to stick? What is the pathway from the comment being made to the belief forming in the person's mind?

In some cases, it may be that the person already had some sort of preoccupation or dissatisfaction. They may have convinced themselves that yes, maybe there was an issue, but they had rationalised it by thinking that nobody else could see it, and they tried hard not to let it bother them too much. So, you can imagine the impact it would have had when they realised that actually, somebody else could see it too, because then their view of themselves would change.

The alternative possibility is that it wasn't something Chloe had particularly thought about before. It might be something she was vaguely aware of, or it might not have crossed her mind at all. She was quite happy with the status quo and then someone innocently asks, 'What's wrong with your neck?' Suddenly, she feels horrible. It's that pit of the stomach feeling that you get when something really shakes you to the core. We all know what that feels like. And in this situation, she immediately links that specific experience of someone commenting on an aspect of her appearance with that horrible, gut-wrenching feeling. The intensity of that experience creates the belief and feelings that her appearance is abnormal.

## TRYING TO AVOID HUMILIATION

Having this experience and going on to develop body dissatisfaction or BDD may be hard for people to understand. So, let's look at it in a different way. Chloe enjoys writing, so let's say she wrote something she was proud of, and posted it online. Now, imagine that the feedback she got back was mostly negative, that she was belittled and humiliated for her work. She would never want to experience that level of criticism ever again.

So, what does she do? She does what any one of us would do. She avoids posting any more of her writing online and thinks, *I'm not subjecting myself to that kind of experience ever again. It was absolutely, utterly humiliating.* Irrespective of what Chloe thought of her writing, the experience would have eroded her confidence in herself and her work. And she would have stopped writing just to avoid any chance of experiencing the same kind of humiliation again. In addition, every time she had to write something in her job, she would become anxious about what the possible feedback would be, even if she had never been anxious before in that situation. The original experience was so awful, that the fear of being criticised again for her writing has spread into other areas that were not previously a problem for her.

Being singled out for an aspect of your appearance can be even more destabilising. It isn't like hiding your writing from anyone else's inspection. You know that any "flaws" in your appearance that have been pointed out to you are there for all to see, all the time.

Other people's opinions of us matter to us all to some degree. This is normal and it is important to consider the thoughts and feelings of the people in our lives, just as it's important to feel like a part of society. These thoughts play into our concerns about appearance too. That is especially true in adolescence. Adolescence is a difficult life stage at the best of times. Trying to reconcile the expectations of family, friends, peers, and teachers, coping with hormonal changes and finding your place in the world is a constant challenge. With all that going on, your focus on appearance changes. As your hormones kick in, you begin to feel attraction to other people, and you hope that those attractions can be reciprocated. Suddenly the value placed on appearance is much more significant. Suddenly you are being assessed and judged in a different kind of way by people you have known for years.

Chloe didn't know if her feelings were a symptom of growing up or something else. And for many people, the onset of body image issues can be confused by all the other things that are going on in their lives.

In the early stages of the development of body image and BDD, the "objective" appraisal of other people is easier to believe than your own judgements. You may not have any concerns about your physical appearance, but if just one person mentions that your skin looks oily, then it becomes very easy to fixate on that. Later, as body dissatisfaction takes hold, your reality becomes so skewed that you disregard the views of other people, because your own negative self-image is deeply ingrained. So even if one hundred people tell you that your skin looks lovely, you disregard them all on the basis that you assume they are lying, or just trying to be nice.

The idea that her neck looked strange took root very quickly in Chloe. She believed she was a freak. She thought that everyone was looking at her as if there was something abnormal or disgusting about her. For most people with body image issues, that is such an overwhelmingly unpleasant feeling that they decide that they will not ever risk having that feeling again because it was so awful. And they will do anything to prevent experiencing that feeling again by camouflaging or hiding the perceived flaw; they may even stop going out in public at all.

## CAN ONE COMMENT CAUSE BODY IMAGE ISSUES OR BDD?

It is important to clarify that her sister's comment did not give Chloe body image issues. You can take a hundred people and make a comment like that to them without any of them being adversely affected by it, unless they already had low self-esteem. At worst, some of them may have thought, *Oh, maybe I should get that checked out by a doctor*, but because of Chloe's worries about her appearance, the comment exacerbated her anxiety and fuelled the emerging belief that there was something wrong with her.

The fact that someone drew attention to an aspect of Chloe's appearance, irrespective of whether or not that was one of her key concerns, also reinforced the fact that appearance is important, noticeable and judged. In other words, it confirms what we all know: appearance does matter. But of course, it matters to us all in different ways, and becomes more or less important at different times of our lives. It isn't just an issue of wanting to appear attractive; people may wish to look distinctive, professional, or unconventional, so our perception of our own appearance can shift.

Concerns about appearance aren't shallow. In fact, the importance of appearance has its roots way back in history with our earliest ancestors. Their life was tough, and their survival was only possible so long as they were part of a wider community. But if they were considered hideous, diseased, or badly injured, they would not be able to find a mate, they would not be able to contribute to the survival of the community, and ultimately they would be rejected from the tribe. Left alone in a hostile environment, without food, friendship, or protection, they would face a very uncertain future and would be less likely to survive.

It's amazing how many of the feelings we still experience today come down to us from our caveman forebearers – we've already mentioned anxiety and how the feelings of anxiety we experience today are just the same as the adrenaline-fuelled response to danger that they had.

From an evolutionary perspective, we are still programmed to react with fear in cases where we feel like we may be about to be kicked out of our tribe, i.e. rejected. It is in our DNA, and part of our instinct to survive.

What does rejection mean today? It may mean being cut out of family groups, or being excluded by friendship groups. Humans are social animals, and rejection can lead to social isolation and loneliness. It can damage self-esteem, leading to depression, high levels of anxiety, and even physical illness.

For all these reasons, concern over one's physical appearance is understandable. It's absolutely normal to have a healthy level of interest in what we look like. As people, we strive to be happy – and that means learning to be content with how we look and feel.

So let's be clear that we're not suggesting an interest or focus on your appearance is wrong. We're not saying you shouldn't care about your appearance. We're just saying that the level of preoccupation that someone suffering with BDD or body image issues has can ruin their life.

Recovering from body image issues does not mean you'll be discouraged from placing any importance on your appearance. It means developing a more balanced view of your appearance, and learning to see yourself as a complete person.

**Your appearance is an important part of who you are, but you are not defined by appearance alone.**

# CHAPTER 5

# WHAT BDD WAS LIKE FOR ME

 *Chloe:* Can you ever get past BDD and body image issues? Once you've had them, how can you ever look at yourself in a non-BDD way ever again?

My body dysmorphia was all-consuming. At its worst, there was no let-up, no going easy on myself, no off days. The hours I spent examining my face and my neck in the mirror changed the way I look at myself for ever. After all of that, I'm not sure you can ever go back to looking at yourself without prejudice. Even now, when I look in the mirror, I don't know if I'm seeing myself with objective eyes.

Now at least I can rationalise it; I can confront my thoughts without automatically assuming that every thought is a true reflection of reality. But at my worst, I would look at myself with revulsion. When I checked on my appearance, it looked as if my face was so enlarged that I could see all my flaws in minute detail. It was almost like there was a spotlight on each imperfection. My skin seemed so bumpy and my pores so large that I just couldn't understand how anyone could look at me with a straight face.

Then I'd go through each of my perceived flaws and peer at them for ages and ages, just trying to find some way of making them seem less obvious, or look for an angle that I could hold my head where the flaw didn't seem quite so horrible. I used to look at a line on my forehead – fortunately it doesn't bother me so much any more – but I would stare and stare at it. I'd move it up and down and study it in detail, from every possible angle, desperately trying to find some light or perspective that would make it a little less objectionable.

It's just like working through a list. You go through every flaw, every single thing you hate about your face and body, one by one. You expose every negative thing. There's nothing positive, and no sense of even trying to be positive. That's not what it's about. It's all extreme damage limitation. And you're working with a list of flaws that only ever gets bigger. Sometimes you'll see an entirely new flaw and wonder how you ever missed it.

Going out would only heighten my anxiety. My parents and my sister were the only people I wouldn't get fully made up around. If I went out, I would have to wear a heavy level of make-up to try to mask some of the flaws. I had to reach a certain level of acceptability for myself and other people, or else I couldn't go out.

I knew I would have to subject myself to everyone's attention. So I'd stand there and stare at myself, wondering how people could even look at me without laughing or grimacing. If I ever stood by a long mirror, I'd study myself from every angle and check my posture. In more recent years, I was looking to see how badly my neck stuck out.

My neck is probably the thing that still gets me most. It's hard to describe it exactly – but to me, it looks like I have a roll of fat on the back of my neck, like a hump. I'm pretty sure it's all because of bad posture. But that's not surprising. For years, I had walked with my shoulders hunched, my face pointing towards the ground. How else could I get through the day without seeing everyone staring at me? I spent hours googling body dissatisfaction issues and comparing my appearance with people online. I found some videos online saying that if you hold your neck in a certain position, it will grow fat to protect the muscle. So I think that's what's happened. I'd look at my neck from every angle and stand by the mirror and try to see how I could change it.

In daylight, I'd really notice the hair on my face. I know everyone has hair on their face, but the more I looked, the more obvious it was. It looked as if my face was covered in this white peach fuzz. I'd try to smooth it down, just to make it a little less obvious. Then I'd check the mole on the side of my face. I hated it, and the thick black hair that grew out of it. So I had to make sure that wasn't too obvious as well. Then there were the blackheads. I'd go right up to the mirror and check my nose and try to see how obvious they were – what exactly could other people see when they looked at me? Then the voice would start up in my head. 'I told you so! I told you it was obvious to everyone. People can see how ugly you are.' And as I looked, it was if a spotlight was shining on everything I hated, magnifying the problem a hundred times. Then I'd circle back and examine all the flaws again and again, until I literally couldn't bear to look at myself any longer.

It was a methodical process. I'd try to establish the best way to stand so that I could look my best if I met someone new. Of course, "the best" was never really acceptable. It wasn't "best" in the sense that it made me happy at all. It was just the least terrible version of myself that I could get away with.

And then I'd look at the opposite extreme – what was the worst I could look? I needed to know so that I could stop standing in a certain way, or try to avoid wearing certain things. I knew I had to cover up my neck, so I started wearing a scarf, but even that wasn't 100% reliable. I had to make sure that it covered the right part of my neck from every possible angle. And then I had to check it – and adjust it. And check it again, and adjust it again. And on and on …

It was a horrible, tiring, depressing ritual. It would really upset me. And it was never enough. So later, I'd go back and check again to see if there was any difference in my appearance from before – or if anything had got worse. There was a real difference between daylight and artificial light too. Artificial light masked some of the problems, but daylight was totally unforgiving. So that's when I tried to do most of my checking; I wanted to get what I thought was the most honest representation possible.

And then, after all the checking, I'd spend hours researching how to get rid of blackheads, how to make blemishes smaller, how to make my skin smoother …

I could never work out why nobody ever said anything to me. Why didn't anyone take me to one side and tell me they could see all the flaws? I started questioning their perspective too; I had to bend the truth to fit my version of events – that I was a hideously ugly person. And that is an exhausting way to live.

From speaking to Lauren and Annemarie, I know I was trying to read people's minds, to figure out what they were thinking. This is a problematic thinking style. Immediately upon meeting someone my mind would divert from what they were saying to me, to what they were probably thinking when they looked at me. One glance was all it took to make me assume that they thought I was ugly. That would then feed back into my belief that I was ugly. And the longer I spent with an individual, the more I'd interpret their behaviour as proof of how hideous I was. I would take that as evidence that I was ugly, and I would mull it over in my head.

Still to this day, I find it hard not to fall back into mind reading. Either I wonder what people are thinking, or I project my thoughts onto them. I'm still working hard to try to overcome the urge to assume that every thought that comes into my head is automatically true. It is hard work, but the techniques I've learnt are effective. You will learn more about the techniques Lauren and Annemarie taught me in Part II.

BDD is such a socially crippling illness that it makes living a normal life virtually impossible. When you are so consumed by the pain and anxiety of BDD, you've got nothing left to give. The little everyday things that most people take for granted feel 10 times more difficult. The time and effort it takes to get ready – just to leave the house – make life utterly exhausting.

One of the hardest things was trying to be "normal" around other people. I remember one time when my sister suggested going to Brighton the day after our birthday with her boyfriend and a mutual friend. But lots of people were coming around to celebrate our birthday with us, and I knew I'd need the next day to recover. So I made sure everyone knew I wouldn't be able to go to Brighton; I told them over and over again, but then the next day everyone tried to persuade me to go anyway.

Afterwards, my friend wrote me a letter saying I really needed to put more effort into our friendship, and I was stunned. I didn't know what else I could have done. It hurt so much knowing that people couldn't understand. Why did they think I would turn down a day at the seaside with the people I loved, unless I was really suffering?

I felt like I hardly had any friends left – and I wouldn't ever be able to make any more. The more difficult my life got, the more I retreated into myself. I knew that if this was as good as my life was ever going to get, there wasn't any point going on. I knew I wouldn't ever achieve anything meaningful in my life. And if I looked ahead five years, I wasn't even sure if I would still be around. If I made it past my twenty-first birthday, I assumed I'd be living with my parents, locked inside, day after day after day. Not doing anything. Not achieving anything. Wasting away. Getting through a single day was hard enough, so I didn't know how on earth I was going to manage another year, or however more years I still had to come.

If I got into a fight with Olivia or my friends, it could get really personal. I knew they were only trying to motivate me, but it didn't help. For me the worst part was knowing that all the things they said about me were true. That was one time when it wasn't so good to have a twin sister – she was moving on, doing the things girls our age did. But I wasn't. And I believed that I was always going to be a burden on our family.

I felt like the secret family member – the one that no one ever really talked about. I literally felt like the Hunchback of Notre Dame. There's a song he sings – 'Out There' – when he's up in the bell tower looking down at all the people living their lives, saying they don't know how lucky they are. I felt like that. I wondered how it would be to have just one normal day. What would that feel like? I just wanted one more chance to do normal things, to go to everyday places and speak to people without feeling like a freak. I listened to that song a lot.

As soon as the anxious thoughts and worries crashed in, they would start to escalate and make me feel even worse. Lauren called it worst-case scenario thinking, which is being trapped into thinking that the worst-case scenario will happen in every situation. The problem is that once you start thinking like this, it's very hard to stop.

That is what living with BDD was like for me. This is how it feels when you're so wracked with BDD and depression that you can't do anything ... And because you don't do anything, you get even more depressed ... And that makes the social anxiety even worse. It's a constant spiral of negative thinking and feelings – once you've unpeeled one level, you have to address the next one. Living like that isn't really living in any real sense. And that is what I would like to tell people when they say, 'BDD – oh, that's just vanity isn't it?'

I started to sleep a lot. I couldn't cope with the reality of my life and sleeping was just my way of shutting off the negative thoughts and worries, and not having to feel the anxiety and depression. It was an avoidance tactic, a safety behaviour – I know that now.

I thought my way of looking at myself and the world would never change. I thought my life was over.

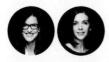 ***Lauren and Annemarie:*** It is the unhelpful, and usually untrue, beliefs about our bodies and they way we think people will react to us that lie at the heart of body image problems and BDD.

Just to clarify, thoughts can often be referred to as beliefs – they are both types of cognition. So when we discuss challenging thoughts and beliefs, we're referring to the things that you think about or believe, as well as your assumptions or interpretations. However, we also use these terms to refer to different types of cognitions – thoughts, beliefs, interpretations, and assumptions – as they all have slightly different features.

For example, beliefs are usually more entrenched and stuck, whereas thoughts are more fluid and come and go frequently. Confused? Don't worry, we talk about this more in Part II. But essentially, if you are not sure whether it is a belief, or a thought, or an assumption, don't worry! The same strategies to challenge our unhelpful cognitions can be applied to all of them just as effectively.

## WHAT ARE YOUR UNHELPFUL BELIEFS ABOUT YOURSELF AND YOUR APPEARANCE?

It is important to identify what your unhelpful beliefs and thoughts are if you want to change them. We have a number of ways of doing this. Here's a quick question to get you started:

If you went to live on a desert island, do you think you would still worry about your appearance? If you say yes, then it's very likely that your self-perception – how you see and feel about your body – is a major problem for you.

But if you say no, then it's more likely that your key unhelpful beliefs are about what other people think about you and your appearance.

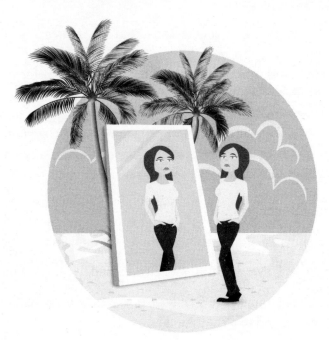

Questions like this help us figure out some of the key unhelpful beliefs in your body image problems. We will help you try to work out what your main unhelpful beliefs are about yourself and your appearance in Part II.

## HOW HAVE YOUR BELIEFS DEVELOPED?

With Chloe, we spent some time finding out why she would ever think she was so freakishly ugly. Sometimes if a person can understand how their beliefs have developed, it can help them to understand that they are accepting a skewed version of reality, not an objectively accurate reality. While this can be a very helpful process for some people, it is not necessary helpful for all people with body image issues. Sometimes we can isolate a defining feature from their past, or a collection of experiences that have made them vulnerable to developing body image issues or BDD. But sometimes, a body image issue has appeared recently (e.g. after a traumatic experience, or specific situation) and we only need to focus on how the problem presents itself now to help resolve the issue.

It can be helpful to think of these past events or experiences as "emotional injuries" complete with "emotional bruises". When we suffer a physical injury, we develop bruises when the blood vessels under the skin rupture. Although bruises heal over time, the point of injury may remain sensitive, or require physiotherapy and other treatment to heal properly. Before it heals, the bruise will remain sensitive when pressure is applied, reminding us that we have to be careful while the injury is still healing.

We can think of body image issues in the same way. Something may have happened in the past (e.g. a comment about your weight 10 years ago) that left a psychological and emotional injury. You might not feel the injury all the time, but a current event (e.g. someone mentioning their own weight loss and recommending their latest diet) can press on that sensitive spot and really hurt you. It's like an emotional bruise caused by anxiety, shame, or embarrassment. Like any underlying injury, it may not always be noticeable, or you may forget about it for a while, but at some point there will be pressure applied and it will result in emotional pain. These emotional bruises are clues to what your underlying beliefs about yourself and your appearance may be, so if you notice an emotional bruise, it might be helpful to note it down. You'll be able to work on that belief in Part II when we talk about changing beliefs.

## THINKING PROBLEMS

We are all bombarded with thoughts every day: interesting, happy, sad, strange, and sometimes downright weird thoughts. With body image issues, it isn't just the thoughts themselves that are the problem – it is what you take the thoughts to actually mean about yourself. So, we're looking for patterns in the way you think to help you identify these unhelpful thoughts and meanings. For example, you might see someone very attractive on the train and you think about how beautiful they are. On its own, that thought isn't damaging, but you might then go on to think that because they are beautiful, they must have an easy life and that means that your life can never compare with theirs. Consequently, you believe you'll never be as happy as they are. Now you can see that this has become a very damaging train of thought. We would call this Predicting the Future and Worst Case Scenario or Catasrophising-type thinking. We will teach you to identify these thinking styles and label them, which again will help you change them to more adaptive and helpful ways of thinking.

## WHY ARE THESE THOUGHTS SO CONVINCING?

Why do the things you believe about your appearance feel true? It is usually because the emotion that you experience in relation to those beliefs is so strong that it makes you think that the beliefs must be true. An example of that is somebody who thinks they are overweight. They are so convinced of this fact that they doubt the evidence to the contrary. One patient swore that she was a size 16, but then, when we looked at the label in her jeans, it confirmed that she was wearing size 10. She didn't believe that could possibly be true, in spite of the evidence to the contrary, so she decided that the label must be wrong.

But how can her belief be so strong, even when the evidence proves it is incorrect?

This is an example of a thinking problem called Emotional Reasoning, which refers to basing things on how you feel, not on reality. You feel that because the emotion is intense, the belief must be true, e.g. 'I feel that I am hideous, therefore it must be true.'

The problem is that all the evidence in the world isn't more persuasive than your own feelings. Your innate feeling will always seem more credible to you. So, gathering evidence to the contrary is just a starting point. You then have to challenge the belief in more detail, and understand that despite how you feel, your initial belief might not be true and that there is an alternative way of seeing things that fits with the evidence.

## CHALLENGING YOUR UNHELPFUL THOUGHTS AND BELIEFS

Challenging the way you think is a very important part of the treatment process, and as therapists we use different strategies to help someone identify and change their unhelpful thoughts, worries, and beliefs.

The first thing we'll do is help you to identify what your beliefs are so that you can spot them more easily. This is a process called self-monitoring – and we'll guide you through it in Part II. Once you are able to identify your thoughts you can identify the thinking problems and then begin to challenge them, using some really effective cognitive strategies and experiments. One such strategy is a technique that Chloe found really useful, called the Two Hands Thinking Technique. This will help you confront and challenge your unhelpful thoughts in a completely different way. We'll tell you everything you need to know about the Two Hands Thinking Technique in Part II.

# CHAPTER 6

# CHANGING MY THINKING

*Chloe:* If I had to put a figure on it, I would have said that my appearance was on my mind at least six hours of the day when I was out of the house. If you have experienced BDD or body image issues yourself, you'll understand what that does to your daily life.

I was so conscious of my appearance that I would have to check how I looked at least 20 times a day to make sure I had done as much as I could to camouflage my flaws. If I couldn't find a mirror, I would use any reflective surface I could find. It didn't feel like a simple urge or an itch. It was a compulsion, a growing sense of unease that I couldn't ignore. And it was so deeply ingrained that I still have to fight the urge to do it now.

The checking was quite low key at first, but escalated quickly. It didn't just take up my time, it consumed my energy. When I wasn't checking, I was already thinking about where and when I was going to be able to check again, or worrying about how my appearance might have altered since I last checked.

By this point in my story I had dropped out of college altogether, and Mum and Dad were getting more and more worried that the daughter that had once been happy, confident, and loving had withdrawn from the world. I still liked seeing very close family, but it was embarrassing hearing about all the things they were doing when I wasn't doing anything. I couldn't just tell them I'd been spending my days hiding from the world in my bed. So eventually, I stopped seeing them too. Extended family members would wonder why they hadn't seen me and no one had any good answers for them.

Even in my darkest hours, I still felt pangs of guilt. I knew that I was making Mum and Dad's lives harder, and I would have done almost anything to try to please them, or at least give them a glimmer of hope. So I finally caved in, and on their suggestion, started looking for a part-time job. The thought terrified me, but for my own sake too, I knew I had to try. There was already a big gap on my CV where my A Levels should be, and no likelihood of filling that gap with any other qualifications.

I managed to get a shelf-stacking job in Tesco (a supermarket / grocery store) on a Saturday. It was a daunting prospect, a bit like starting out at school all over again. So many people worked there and a lot of them were around my age, but infinitely more confident in their own skin. It must have been obvious that I found interacting with them difficult, and I hoped I just came over as shy rather than rude or standoffish.

I kept my head down, just like in school, but it was really difficult and I nearly quit a few weeks in. But I'd only lasted a few weeks in my last part-time job, and I knew I couldn't do that again. Somehow, I found the strength to keep going. Something – probably the fear of how another failed job was going to look on my CV – kept me going, and I stuck it out. I know it was only a day a week, but after living such a secluded life, and only ever seeing my own family, suddenly being surrounded by thousands of people in the space of a day was mind blowing.

I was lucky in a way, because I had such a positive young woman to show me the ropes. She was probably only a year or two older than me, but so different, so relaxed. Whereas I was always scared of getting something wrong, she didn't care. She would just have a laugh with the boss. We were like chalk and cheese really, but I don't think I could have survived as long as I did if it hadn't been for her. I felt okay when she was around. And I took my lead from her.

I couldn't wear a scarf but I was given a shirt with a high collar and a fleece which came up quite high – and I was just about okay with that. I still had to do a lot of checking in the mirror on my breaks. I would spend 15 minutes or more in the bathroom at a time, and as soon as anyone came in, I'd just pretend I was washing my hands. And I would have little tricks, like pretending I was going to the loo again, just so I knew there'd be enough time to check everything a certain amount of times.

The lighting was really horrible in there so I had to lean right over the sink to get close enough to the mirror to be able to see everything. I'd turn my head to the side and check my neck. Because I didn't have a scarf on, I'd take my hand and put it on my neck to try to push it in and flatten it as much as possible. I was sure that people could see all my facial hair, so I would turn my head from side to side and try to flatten that down as much as possible. I had to check if there were any red patches on my face, because it was quite physical work, and I didn't want it to look as if my skin tone was horribly uneven. If I thought I had any dry skin or patches, I would try to get rid of them as best I could.

When I was checking, I wasn't thinking that I was going to be able to make any dramatic improvements. I was really only trying to get to a level that's ... okay is not the word ... I had to get it to the stage where it wasn't mortifying. I made sure I did all the face stuff first, do the neck a couple of times and then just have one last check in the mirror, as closely as possible, so I could really see my pores.

I couldn't have any make-up with me, and I didn't have a locker, so I couldn't take anything to help me. That was hard. And it was tiring having to spend so much time in between shifts relentlessly checking myself, and then subject myself to the scrutiny of so many people. I was utterly exhausted by the end of the day.

A lot of people liked the girl I was working with and talked about how attractive she was. But I didn't want to be judged on my looks, negatively or positively. I didn't want anyone to say anything at all – so that made me even more self-conscious. As soon as I heard the comments going around – hearing that so-and-so likes so-and-so, I thought, *Oh, no! People are paying attention to appearance*. When you're in an environment like that, you know that everyone is being judged on the basis of their appearance, consciously or not.

Although I did a lot of work behind the scenes, I did have to interact with customers too. I'd never been in such a busy environment before – particularly in the run-up to Christmas – and that was extremely difficult. It took me a long time to get used to where everything was in the shop. Fortunately, we had a badge helpfully pointing out that I was new to the team, so I was grateful for that. If someone asked me a question, I wasn't confident enough to look them in the eye. I didn't want to see them looking at me, so I had to look slightly over their shoulder instead. I certainly didn't want anyone saying I was rude, so I dreaded customer interactions and difficult customers.

I automatically assumed nobody liked me because I was quiet. But I'd always been that way. So I didn't look forward to going to work at all; I did it more for my parents. And I worried about it constantly. All of it. Every single aspect of working in that shop worried me. I wouldn't sleep very well on a Friday night, and I had really bad anxiety before going in on Saturday. And then when I got home again, I needed all of the Sunday to recover.

Mum and Dad knew it was difficult, but they saw the job as a useful distraction for me. But if they thought that having a part-time job was going to help me recover, they were going to be disappointed. Despite constantly feeling like I wanted to leave, I kept on giving it one more week, one more week …

Around the same time I started at Tesco, I was referred to a clinical psychologist. And as she was actually a specialist in BDD, I finally felt like I might be getting somewhere. I had about nine sessions, but then she went on maternity leave, and I was scared that history was going to repeat itself. I felt like I was going to find myself right back at the start of the process, unable to make any more progress. But before she left, she suggested I get in touch with Lauren Callaghan.

By then I was wary about seeing another specialist. I didn't know if I had the energy to tell my life story again, but I started seeing Lauren in November 2013, and quickly built up a good rapport with her. In time, I realised that this last change of circumstances had actually been a blessing in disguise.

To begin with, Lauren quickly proved to me that I could trust her, and that made it easier to make progress. She talked to me about exposure therapy. But unlike last time, we worked up to it gradually. She broke it down into smaller steps to make it feel so much more manageable for me. She didn't push me or force me to take on more than I could manage. But neither did she sit back and wait for things to happen.

Above all, Lauren made me feel understood. I think that was the first time in my life that I had ever felt like somebody genuinely knew what I was going through. When you have lived your life feeling alone and different, that makes a huge difference.

It wasn't po-faced though. I was able to have a laugh with Lauren, and later with Annemarie. That might not seem like a big deal, but when you've been hiding away from so much of life, having people around you that you can relax with, even when talking about BDD, is invaluable.

It wasn't all straightforward. Just getting the train to see Lauren was a challenge in itself, so we broke it down into smaller activities, so that instead of trying to cope with the vast idea of a trip to London, I approached it in more manageable steps.

The train trip became a part of my exposure therapy too and we'd talk about it when I got to my appointment. Lauren helped me to see that I could carry on challenging my unhelpful beliefs and safety behaviours even without her being there, and that really helped me to get maximum value from our time together. (And then, as I started to get a little bit more confident, Lauren would ask me to travel to my appointment without my scarf on.)

As promised, the exposure therapy we did together started very gently. Initially, Lauren would ask me to think about things in the safety of my own home – little, manageable things, perhaps tying my hair up in the house and then popping outside with it still tied up.

And then, during the session, she asked if it would be okay to take my scarf off – just for a minute or two – and we'd talk about the experience of doing it. Gradually, we would extend the time and discuss what made it bearable – knowing it was going to end – and how I felt about it. I knew that if she asked me to do something, Lauren would be prepared to do it too. So if she asked me to come to a session without any make-up on, she wouldn't wear any either. When I needed a little bit of a push, she said we'd just do a little bit and see how it went.

To begin with, we used to go out on to the street and just walk up and down together. That was all. And then, if I felt ready, I'd take off my scarf and we'd walk up and down again. Just for a few minutes. Then I'd put my scarf back on. These little bursts of exposure were so small – and so controlled – that I was able to talk to Lauren and reflect on my feelings at every stage of the process, so I could register the changes in my emotional state. And if anything felt like too big a step, Lauren would just break it down into smaller steps.

As we walked, Lauren would ask me how it felt and we'd discuss my thought processes – it really was nothing like the kind of exposure therapy I'd experienced before. Last time we had just done it, and we hadn't talked about my thoughts or feelings at all. We also challenged my thinking, and in Part II, you'll read about the Two Hands Thinking technique, which was very useful for me in coming up with new ways to think about things. We also identified my safety behaviours and worked on more productive ways to respond.

It was still difficult work, but I didn't mind because I could see and feel how this was going to help me. With Lauren guiding me through it, step by step, I felt like I was working towards something positive. Long-term goals were too distant, too hard – so it was nice to have little goals that I could genuinely work towards in the here and now.

The exposure therapy was more gradual, so that when I did start establishing eye contact with people, it felt a bit more natural. It wasn't suddenly forced on me. Of course, I was still very nervous, but by that point I had built up a good rapport with Lauren. I genuinely trusted her and she explained the processes we were following in a way that made sense. I didn't have to stare at anyone or hold their gaze; it was just a case of looking at someone to see if they were looking at me and then looking away. That way it didn't feel like a horribly unnatural process.

Walking along the busy and bustling London Bridge was obviously a very different experience to fixating on people in an empty village street too, so it didn't feel quite as forced. When I started looking around, I noticed that people weren't staring at me. And the more we did it, the easier it became to reverse some of my ingrained thinking that everyone was staring at me in revulsion.

The whole process with Lauren and Annemarie was like a series of "lightbulb moments". It occurred to me that maybe people weren't paying as much attention to me as I'd thought. Of course, it didn't transform my life overnight – as soon as someone looked back, I still thought, *Here we go, they're staring!* But Lauren would rationalise it, saying, 'Yes, they looked when they saw you looking, but then they looked away. They didn't stare and their expression didn't change. Or they just glanced and looked away – it's a natural, human thing to glance around and meet someone's gaze.'

I started to understand my brain's processes a bit more. I saw that my brain was taking information and distorting it into my own personal ideology. It's interesting how your personal filter works. If someone wasn't looking at me, I didn't take that as evidence to counterbalance my view of events, and I didn't take it as cause to start questioning my beliefs. So with Lauren's help, I started to practise operating on a more objective level.

I think that was the first time I became aware of just how ingrained my thinking was – and how forceful and powerful it was. When I was unwell with BDD there wasn't any flexibility in my thinking, it was all very categorical – I was ugly and that was all there was to it. I couldn't really see the other side of the argument. I couldn't believe that people weren't looking at me. So it was a difficult process, like exercising a mental faculty that had been dormant for so long, but I knew it was necessary for me to get to grips with a different perspective.

## FACING YOUR FEARS

 *Lauren and Annemarie:* As you have read in Chloe's story, once you have come up with new ways of thinking about your body image concerns, we then test out these new interpretations with experiments. We need to see if your new way of thinking about things fits with reality – so we put it to the test. In cases where anxiety is the predominant emotion, as it is in BDD and body image problems, this is called Exposure Therapy – and it means exposing you to situations which are anxiety-provoking. We need to make sure it's a fair experiment so that we can use the results to either confirm or dismiss our new interpretation. That means doing it without any of your safety behaviours.

## Sound scary?

That's because you're so used to avoiding these anxiety-provoking triggers, or using safety behaviours to get through them, that the prospect of facing situations without any of the things you did to reduce the anxiety, or to avoid it, is scary. However, as Chloe explained, when you start to accept that maybe there is another way to see things, then it gets easier to take that first step and test things out in an experiment. And don't worry, you won't have to do the scariest thing first – you build up to it, bit by bit, with smaller experiments.

Also, it is important to know that even if rationally you have accepted that your feared outcome is not likely to come true, and that there is an alternative way of thinking about things, you might still feel very anxious in these situations. Why is that? Well, by now your body is conditioned to react with fear to these triggers. It's got used to it. Also, there will always be a little part of you saying, 'What happens if what I worry about really does come true?' Even if you're almost certain it won't!

So until you do the experiments, you're still going to feel anxious in these situations. But don't worry, this anxiety will start to subside in a process that we call habituation. We'll discuss this in more detail in Part II.

In Chloe's case, she was worried that people would notice her neck and how deformed (she thought) it was, so she used to avoid being seen in public without using her scarf to hide her neck. When she bought into the idea that perhaps her neck wasn't deformed, and that people might not be looking at it, she felt brave enough to start testing out whether this new way of thinking might be true.

We came up with a graduated plan for Chloe to reach her ultimate goal of not having to wear her scarf, or any other form of camouflage, in public. As Chloe explained, she had to get the train to come and see us. So we agreed a series of experiments with the ultimate aim that Chloe would travel on the train without wearing her scarf. At first Chloe travelled with her mum to make the journey less stressful. But on subsequent trips, her mum sat in a different place, and then stopped going altogether. In fact, this happened quite quickly and it only took three sessions before Chloe could travel into central London (which is very, very busy) on her own!

Given that she could barely leave the house before she started her sessions with us, that was a pretty amazing achievement. We then set some experiments for Chloe to try while she was travelling. She started by taking off her scarf while she waited on the station platform, and then put it back on when she got on the train. As she got more confident, she started to leave it off for a few stops, and then eventually, she was able to travel all the way to London, on a very busy train, without her scarf or any new or compensatory safety behaviours – such as sitting in a different area of the train so no one could see her, or wearing a coat with large collars.

Another thing about experiments is that they are not predetermined. We do not know the outcome – so it is an excellent way to gather information and check out what is happening in reality (not in your forecasted worries). Even if the experiment doesn't go perfectly, it still helps challenge the unhelpful belief that things will be horrific and that you won't cope. Sometimes, experiments do throw up unusual outcomes, but this gives us a chance to think about unusual outcomes too, and the reasons why they arise. (It won't necessarily be because you are ugly or that people are shocked by your appearance.)

Let's look at another example involving Chloe. As you know, she believed that everyone was looking at her in a funny way and thought she was hideous. So the first thing we challenged is the belief that somebody would look at her like that, and think she was ugly, using our Two Hands Thinking Technique. Then, once we came up with a new way of thinking about things, we put it to the test ...

We went out together and asked Chloe to stop people and ask them for directions. We deliberately chose a common scenario – people stop people in the street to ask for directions all the time – so it didn't feel like an unusual thing for her to do.

In this scenario, we were confronting the worries that people might stare at her, say something rude about her appearance, or look at her in disgust. We found that, out of ten people, three of them helped us by giving us the right directions; four of them tried to help but sent us in the wrong direction, two people ignored us altogether, and one person didn't even understand what we were asking. So each time we had a different outcome, with most people stopping to help and give us directions, without looking shocked by Chloe's appearance. Only two people out of ten ignored us, and we reasoned that this was because they were too busy to stop, or were too self-involved to notice us! Overall, the experiment showed us that, in a real situation, people didn't react in horror when they saw Chloe. In fact, most people were very helpful.

What conclusions do we draw from this? That it is not Chloe's appearance that is the problem here. The real problem was her worrying about her appearance and scrutinising herself.

In Part II, you will also learn new ways to interpret events using the Two Hands Thinking Technique. This is what helped Chloe challenge the belief that people thought she was ugly when they looked at her. When you can do this, you too will be able to do the exposure experiment and reassess your beliefs. We're going to give you all the tips and tools you need to carry out your own experiments in Part II.

# CHAPTER 7

# FIGHTING BACK AGAINST BDD

*Chloe:* Therapy isn't a wand-waving cure; changing your thinking is hard work. There is a lot of harm to undo.

Lauren once told me that reinforcing a negative idea in your mind and making it stick can happen very quickly. For various reasons, my mind very easily accepted the idea that my neck looked strange, and I stared consolidating that belief almost straightaway.

Reversing such a firmly held belief was going to take time, and it was harder to combat it without Lauren there; I couldn't tell my mum about the unhelpful thoughts that popped into my head and discuss them objectively with her! So it took time for me to feel like I could capture my negative thoughts and assess them objectively. I'm much better at doing it now, but if I go out and I'm feeling vulnerable, I find it very easy to slip back into old patterns, and I walk with my eyes to the ground. If I try to look up and see someone glancing at me, the same old voice starts up again. If I hear laughter it immediately springs to mind that they're laughing at me. Those automatic negative thoughts are still there – I know that everyone has negative thoughts – but the difference now is that I know how to respond to them ...

It's like rewinding a coil; I track the thought back and confront it by saying, 'No, you don't have any basis for believing that thought.' But I do feel like the more I do it, the easier it gets – and the better I get at it. I realise that my negative settings are so ingrained that there is still a lot of work ahead of me. But I also know that, as my self-image and self-worth go on improving, it'll go on getting easier.

I have found myself slipping into that process more naturally now, but its effectiveness is partly down to my mood. Truly believing that my first assumption is not the correct assumption is harder if I'm feeling low. In the past, there were times when things happened that really upset me, but I'd be far too upset to confront them at the time. So I would go back to them and replay them over and over in my head, and try to reflect on what had happened. Lauren encouraged me to stop that. So as I started to feel better, I made myself confront things as soon as possible after the event. And now I know that doing that makes it so much easier to challenge and rationalise my thoughts before I can try to catastrophise what has happened.

When I'm out and about, I try to walk taller and straighter. My posture has been bad for so long that it seemed really unnatural at first and it made me feel a bit tense. But again, Lauren encouraged me to glance around a bit, and just try to take things slowly. Annemarie also told me how important it was to regulate my breathing – and that was so much easier when I walked with my head held high. It gives me more of an opportunity to take in my surroundings too, so I look at things more and slow down, especially in London, when there are so many interesting things to see.

Within a few weeks of seeing Lauren, I started wearing my scarf less and less. To start with, I'd only wear it five days a week instead of seven. And I kept cutting that number down. Obviously, I do still wear a scarf if it's genuinely cold, but I try very hard not to wear it in situations that I don't need it. I agreed times with Lauren when I wouldn't wear a scarf or clothes with a high neckline. She developed a little app so that I could record the situation and say how I was thinking and feeling, and then how I responded to the situation. It meant I could always tell her what my responses were in any given situation.

It may not sound very dramatic, but it's surprising how effective lots of little day-to-day improvements can be. I still have the issue with my neck – it hasn't gone away, so I still feel some of the same anxiety. But it's not so ingrained that I think I can't wear something, or I have to wear something with a high collar to cover it up. For a long time, it would totally dictate the clothes that I wore, so I couldn't wear anything with a low neckline. But I don't feel like I'm ruled by that compulsion any more. And I think that one of the secrets of living with BDD is learning to embrace the negative thoughts and carry on without letting them consume you. That sounds simple, but doing it takes time.

Even while you're on the path to recovery, you still have to try to get on with your day-to-day life. I made the trip to see Lauren every week and I continued going to work at Tesco every Saturday. It might not sound like much, but it was a life, of sorts.

As well as my neck, Lauren helped push my tolerance of my body hair issue. I hated how the hair on my arm looked and I shaved it as soon as I felt it was getting too visible. I hadn't really challenged myself like this before, but Lauren asked me if I minded it on my sister. Olivia didn't shave her arms and, like me, the hair was quite dark and quite visible on her arms. But I didn't mind it on her at all. Just on me. So Lauren suggested it would be a good idea to stop shaving my arms – just for a little bit – to see how I coped. She wanted to see how far I could go without shaving and then push myself just a little bit further. And that's what I did. I let the hair on my arms get a little bit longer every time. And every time it got that little bit easier.

As you can probably tell, there wasn't any secret to recovery, and no tricks – just lots of hard work. When I started to work with Annemarie, we did a lot of work on eliminating my bargaining tools. So if I was expecting a difficult day, I would plan to spend the next day in bed to recover. That was my way of coping. It was just a way of offsetting the difficulty of doing something hard. But this strategy was part of the problem – I was too used to making things seem like insurmountable problems.

One of the most useful things I've learnt in sessions is using positive imagery (and we'll cover that in Part II). If I'm feeling heavy and unable to get out of bed, I have to imagine the lightness of my body, and then I break down the process of getting out of bed into smaller steps. When you look at it, getting up in the morning is such a big collection of activities that breaking it down into smaller, more manageable activities makes so much sense. So, for example the first step, if I'm lying down, is literally just to sit up in bed. Then step two would be turning to the side, and step three would be putting my feet on the floor, and so on. But the secret is doing it all slowly and thoughtfully, so that I'm really focusing on the thing I'm doing, not on the next stage.

I didn't realise at first – I would try to do something and it was just too big for me. But I didn't realise I could break it down further still; I could literally break something down into the simplest of things to make it so much more manageable.

Another thing I have to watch is not getting too distracted with things like music and podcasts, because I can easily go into autopilot. It's important that when I'm getting ready, I am absolutely focusing on what I am doing, step by step. So, for example, I need to remember that even small tasks like getting washed are actually made up of lots of little activities, including turning the taps on, using soap, rinsing, and so on – it isn't all one continuous process. I've found that a really useful way of stopping me from feeling overwhelmed by tasks that are too big, and it helps keep my mind grounded in the present. So when I was worrying about my bridesmaid dress fitting, I remembered that I needed to break it down into smaller steps.

Lauren and Annemarie also told me something really important: 'You can always stop it. Whatever it is, whatever you are doing, you can always walk away.' It felt empowering to hear that.

One of the key things I took from a session with Lauren was this: she drew a graph to show how much effort it took for me to do something, compared with how much value

I got out of it. I hadn't thought of activities in those terms before. So I could see that if it took 100% effort to get ready for something that I got just 10% enjoyment out of it, then I believed that perhaps the activity wasn't worth the effort.

Obviously, I knew in my mind that's how I felt, but having a visual representation of it and seeing it logically explained was really helpful. But, I also knew that if I didn't put any effort in, I wouldn't get anything out of it at all, so I realised that it was better to get some enjoyment out of activities than none at all. (That strategy is discussed in Part II, Section 14 – Depression and Medication.)

Breaking things down into smaller and smaller steps has been such an important strategy for me. When you have been struggling for so long trying to handle day-to-day tasks, getting a different perspective on how to do those tasks can be so liberating.

Using the same little-by-little approach, we worked through the process of me wearing less make-up. That was a big thing to tackle. Until then, I literally couldn't go out of the house without wearing make-up – and not in a pop-star kind of way! So it would probably take me a couple of hours to get ready. I just had to wear a certain level of make-up, otherwise no one would be allowed to see me – and there was always the lingering fear that there might be a photo. So tackling that amount of anxiety was an important step forward in helping me get to a stage where I could not only function, but actually leave the house without worrying if I wasn't wearing any make-up.

Lauren and Annemarie worked with me to guard against mind reading – projecting my thoughts when I was talking to people. I always found it frustrating that I never actually managed to get what I wanted to say across in conversations because I was too busy analysing things in my head, looking closely at people's facial features and trying to interpret what their expressions meant. What were they thinking about me? Was it my appearance? Did they think I was weird looking? Did they see something on my face? All those things kept swirling in my mind.

With their help, I began to shift the balance back to focusing on the here and now. Lauren and Annemarie talk more about self-focused attention in Part II.

Recovering from BDD isn't always easy or straightforward. There are times when things definitely feel harder – either with my depression or my BDD – but even then, I feel like I have the tools to cope. It means I've been able to do things I never could have done: two years ago, I couldn't have gone out of the house without make-up, but now – I don't know if okay is the word – but I can do it without thinking about it too much. In my head, I'd rather go out and do something than stay inside, which wasn't the case a few years ago.

For a long time, I always thought about how I could improve myself. Getting used to my actual face – which sounds really strange – was quite challenging. Of course, one of the biggest recent challenges I faced was having the photos taken for this book. When I first went in for the shoot, before I had any make-up on, I was feeling really paranoid. I had to travel up to London with no make-up on which was quite stressful, and then, when I got there, the make-up artist was very pretty and I started comparing myself with her straightaway.

It doesn't necessarily have to be a certain face I want to look like, it's more of an image I want to measure up to in my head. So I was quite nervous that day, and I think a lot of people feel vulnerable when they don't have make-up on. It was daunting sitting there under those glaring vanity lights without any make-up on. But when she finished I was happy – or as happy as possible – with the result. It reminded me a bit of Prom and I felt the same kind of pressure.

But the trick isn't suddenly finding all these high-pressure things easy; it's learning how to cope with them.

I had to pick two images of myself that I liked best, which was difficult. In some of them, I was caught off guard, so that wasn't good either. I certainly didn't like any of the test sheet photos where I had to have a blank face and I looked very strange.

I'm so used to critiquing my image that when I saw the proofs, I immediately started picking out the flaws. I was aware of thinking, *This is what I look like*, but at the same time I couldn't quite believe it. I was worried that people would think I didn't look like I did in my photos.

I think I had such low expectations, but the photos were nicer than I thought they were going to be. I did still have this weird sense that it wasn't me. I know my self-image has been distorted over the years, but seeing myself in a photo can be a bit like an out-of-body experience. When you look in the mirror you see yourself, but how you look in a photo can be very different. It's hard to know which is the real you, but that photo shoot still played its part in helping me process what I actually looked like in a more objective way.

Everyone has told me the photos are really great, and I think they probably show me at the best I can look. Psychologically, it was a big deal. Photos have been such a massive no-no for me for so long that I still find them difficult. But this was another important form of exposure therapy for me. And I think this is a good example of how I can identify opportunities in life for me to practise what I have learnt. So now I know that if I have to have photos taken, I can cope. And coping is such an important thing. It means I can subject myself to situations that I would otherwise shy away from. Being able to endure difficulties without retreating into rumination or self-criticism helps me imagine a brighter future.

Nowadays when I see my friends and they take photos, I just about feel able to be in them too. I still struggle with comparing myself to others sometimes, and I still put people on a pedestal. There are still times when I can't help picking out my own flaws: I can spot the bags under my eyes, or I'll think I can see a double chin, but it no longer dominates my day and I can move on from these thoughts a lot quicker without having to resort to my old safety behaviours.

I still don't know if I can quite look at pictures and accept that it's me without worrying that it's not how I look all the time. But I do at least have a better sense of what I truly look like now, and I've come a long way since ducking out of photos on the way to Alton Towers. Sometimes, I regret that I don't have any photos to document certain times in my life. Most people of my age can look back over the images throughout their life – I can't. And I feel bad for my family and friends if I'm not in their photos. But at the same time, I know that if I did have photos documenting my teenage years, I'd just look back and remember the bad times. It's a double-edged sword really. Now, I just try very hard to balance my own concerns with my thoughts for how other people think and feel.

Looking ahead to Olivia's wedding, I don't think I'm going to try to get out of the photos, because I know that, in the future, I'd be annoyed with myself. And even though my sister has said it would be okay if I don't feel like it, I think she'd be sad. All the other times I've got out of photos, it's been different. It wouldn't have mattered so much. But this time I'm a bridesmaid for my twin sister, so it's different. I know I can go outside of my comfort zone for her.

So I'm looking ahead with more confidence. I know I still have some way to go, but now I know how BDD affects daily life, I've got the tools I need to deal with it. I still wish I'd known about BDD sooner. Not knowing or understanding it was what allowed my BDD to bubble up to crisis point. That's why I like the fact that body image is talked about more in school now; when I was at school there was nothing to educate us. I didn't really know how big an issue it was. I thought it was normal not to like yourself. I thought it was just part and parcel of being a teenager.

If I had the chance, I wish I could tell the teenage Chloe to try to enjoy her teenage years. I was just so scared at secondary school. If I was able to do it again, I'd be so much more self-assured and I'd question everything a lot more.

It sounds strange after everything I've been through, but I could – I should – have been so happy in terms of my physical appearance. I was looking back at photos and I don't understand why I was so self-critical. My own self-worth should have been stronger – and I was good enough to be in my friendship group. I remember Mum saying she hoped I was happy with my Prom photos because she'd be sad if I wasn't. I told her I was happy, even though I wasn't. Things are different now. Now, I'm absolutely fine with them.

Now I finally believe the mantra: *You are okay as you are. You are enough*.

I spent so long wishing for something that was unrealistic and all that time, I was perfectly fine as I was. Actually, I think that was the best I've ever looked! It's a shame I couldn't appreciate it at the time.

I think the fact that I can look at things differently now shows how far I've come. My life has changed in so many ways over the last two years. The single biggest difference is that I'm not scared of depression, anxiety, or BDD. I know how to deal with my feelings. I understand them. They can't hurt me any more. My BDD and anxiety are manageable now. Sometimes I still carry a little mirror around with me, but that doesn't necessarily mean I'll use it as I can choose to use when I want to, not because I feel compelled to check how I look.

I know how to distract myself now if any old BDD habits start creeping back. I can let a destructive thought fade away from my mind.

There will still be times when I don't quite look how I want to look, particularly if I haven't got my make-up quite right, or if I have an idea of how I wanted to look in my head and I don't quite manage to match that ideal. At those times, I might be a bit uncomfortable making eye contact with people. But I sometimes have to remind myself this is still a work in progress. I waited so long for a diagnosis and I had BDD for a long time. But now I'm more aware of how to deal with my feelings – and I can manage the thinking behind them.

I'm aware that my thoughts and feelings are made up of distinct strands that I can untangle and deal with. If my brain goes into mind-reading mode and I start to project thoughts onto other people, part of my brain recognises it straightaway. So I keep telling myself that people aren't looking at me, and even if they are, they're not necessarily thinking anything bad about me. It's good to know that I've got the capacity to do that, as and when I need to. Sometimes I can do it subconsciously now, without it feeling difficult. That's such a big improvement.

Sometimes if I compare myself to people my own age, it makes me want to move ahead faster and faster, because they have jobs and partners. But I just have to remember they didn't have the condition I had. They have had a head start. I didn't go through the same social normalisation process they did, and it's easy to forget that sometimes.

Speaking of improvements, I am seeing them week by week and month by month. I notice that I don't avoid as many social events as I used to. And on days when things are harder, I can at least challenge my thoughts and feelings objectively now, something I wasn't able to do before. It's also good to remind myself of how far I've come. At the moment, you might feel as if you'll never reach that point. But you can.

I was always so jealous of people who could just go out without even thinking about it. It was never like that for me. And if you suffer with BDD or body image problems, you'll know that you have to work 10 times harder than them just to feel like you can be seen in public. But I have also discovered that all that extra effort I have put into my recovery has helped me to appreciate the little things – and life in general – so much more. When you're enjoying the moment, you think back to how you felt before, you remember how bad it was, and it makes you so glad of everything you have now.

As clichéd as it sounds, I know that having gone through this journey, I have a lot of positive experiences to hold on to. And when you've been struggling for so long, they feel even more special. I am so thankful for them, and I'm grateful that I can enjoy the good times in life now.

Will I ever recover from BDD? In my mind, there is an issue with this phrasing, because I feel that saying I am "fully recovered" means that I am back to how I was before all this happened. But I can't un-know what I know now. The experience will always be with me, and it's shaped me as a person. It's a bit like a dormant volcano. I know the BDD is in there somewhere deep inside, but it's sleeping and therefore it's not hurting me. So perhaps I should say that I'm no longer suffering. BDD is no longer a big part of my life. I couldn't have said that even one or two years ago, so I'm happy with that.

I guess it's like an addiction. You have to know your triggers and recognise the signs of relapse if you want to keep your BDD under control. I think that's the key thing with most mental health conditions.

Wherever you are in your battle with body image problems or BDD, I know you can get better. And I know because I've worked through the strategies that Lauren and Annemarie are going to share with you. I didn't think I could live a life free of BDD, but Lauren and Annemarie helped me take a completely different perspective on life.

Thank you for reading my story, and now it's over to you. I really hope you enjoy working through Part II of this book. Your life is going to change in all sorts of positive ways ...

 **_Lauren and Annemarie:_** Chloe spoke a lot about her fear of having photos taken and how she didn't like looking at the results. Certainly photographs, and the expectation that people are going to take photographs, are very big problems for many people with BDD and body image issues. Either people hate photos so much they avoid them completely, or, ironically, they may be so devoted to trying to get a "perfect" photo in which they can minimise their perceived body flaws or imperfections that they take "selfies" in an obsessive way and use them to seek reassurance from others that they look okay. People with body image problems also take photos so they can scrutinise themselves and compare themselves to the image in the photo. As you can see, these are all ways that people with body image issues and BDD reinforce the idea that appearance is everything.

This idea is very difficult to get away from in our current media-driven, instagrammed, "selfie" world, but as we discussed earlier, we need to challenge the idea that your appearance, in this case represented by the photo, is the only important thing about you.

By focusing exclusively on your perceived flaws or imperfections, you're missing so much. The photo was taken to capture that moment in time. It's a record of what you were doing and who you were with, so the meaning is much broader than just your appearance. When you look at the photo you're thinking about the other people, remembering where you were and what you did that day. If you were out walking, it reminds you how much you like walking. If you were on a night out, it reminds you of the good friends you were with.

## LEARNING TO OVERCOME BODY IMAGE PROBLEMS AND BDD

In Part II we'll look at some more techniques to help you. We'll give you a repertoire of methods to apply, as and when you need them.

Bear in mind that change takes hard work – but change is absolutely achievable. Lasting change embeds itself over time, and if you apply these strategies diligently so that they become familiar to you, you'll know that you can rely on them. And knowing that is deeply reassuring.

## WHAT IF MY PROBLEMS COME BACK?

At this point, we just want to mention "relapses" – this refers to times when body image and BDD problems might return to cause you distress all over again. People often worry that if they relapse, they will undo all the good work and find themselves back where they started. This is a very understandable concern for anyone that has fought so hard for so long to get better.

While you can't anticipate every potential problem, we will help you to think about situations that might trigger your body image issues and BDD again, and how to be prepared for this. As you can see from Chloe's story, she occasionally has times when her BDD flares up, but by being proactive and working through these instances, she can stop it from becoming the all-consuming problem it once was. There were times when Chloe accepted that she was preoccupied, and that she allowed things to dominate her more than she should have done. But she got back into the habit of challenging her thoughts in a much more helpful way and was able to get herself back on track. We'll tell you everything you need to know in Part II.

But please bear in mind that ups and downs are inevitable in the recovery process. In other words, there will be times in your journey towards recovery where you feel like you have stalled. At other times you will feel clear momentum, and then you might stall again.

This is because recovery doesn't go in a smooth curve. It's just the same, whether you're recovering from BDD or a physical injury. It takes time. We'll talk more about your recovery progress in Part II so that you know what to do when it seems like your recovery is slowing down.

In our work with Chloe, we encouraged her to do so much of the work herself (just as you will), so that towards the end, she knew exactly what she needed to do. She knew what challenges she needed to embrace and she knew how to enter into new and unfamiliar situations. In short, she knew that she just needed to get on and do it. You will too.

## IT'S YOUR TURN ...

We're so glad you've read Chloe's story. You've seen how she moved from being completely reclusive to building a positive new life for herself. And you can too.

In the next section, we'll guide you through the same process we followed with Chloe. We're going to give you lots to think about – there are experiments to try and new techniques to help you think about your appearance in a more positive way.

We hope you feel excited at the prospect of taking charge of your own recovery, but of course, it's perfectly normal to feel a bit nervous too.

Have faith in yourself. You can do this. The fact that you're reading this book shows that you have the will to get better. Never forget, you have already come a long way.

Good luck with Part II. We look forward to helping you overcome your body image problems and BDD.

# PART II

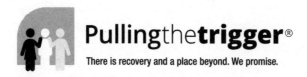

**Pullingthetrigger**®

There is recovery and a place beyond. We promise.

## The Definitive Treatment and Recovery Approach

I felt like I had wasted my youth, that I had let everyone down. Bringing Annemarie and Lauren into my life put me back on track. In just a matter of weeks I could see real progress.

Embrace this approach and embrace your journey. Your recovery is about to begin.

**Chloe Catchpole**

# SECTION 1

# YOUR RECOVERY STARTS HERE

## YOUR BODY IMAGE

Before we begin, it's important to clarify that you may identify with Chloe's story, or parts of it, or you may not relate to it at all. All of those reactions are fine. Body image problems and BDD come in all shapes and sizes, so if your problems are different and you are unsure of whether to continue reading this book, please do. The techniques and strategies we'll be telling you about are for anyone with body image issues or BDD.

In Part I, we introduced the concept of body image to describe the way we think about, feel about, and see our own bodies. Of course, this is a very subjective perception. It starts forming as soon as we become aware of ourselves and we start building up a web of thoughts, feelings, and impressions about our appearance. Our environment and society, family, friends and peers, TV and other media all impact on our sense of identity. These things – and many more – can influence our perception of ourselves and our bodies.

Chloe said that she didn't have a strong sense of her appearance when she was very young. It wasn't really until she went to secondary school and started mixing with people who were more concerned with their appearance that she started forming opinions about her own looks. So, the behaviour of the people she interacted with regularly and how she interpreted their reactions to her appearance had a big impact on her body image.

Our mental picture of how we look is mixed in with our beliefs about our appearance, based on our memories of the things that people have said, and the ways that we believe people have reacted to us when they have met or interacted with us. All those memories and associations can add up to a powerful mix of beliefs about ourselves.

### Body image and felt impressions

We don't use the term body image to describe how you look – our body image is a subjective representation or a felt impression of how we think we look.[6] In other words, this is the picture we have in our minds of our physical appearance. It is based on our existing beliefs about the way we look and how we feel when we look in the mirror, as well as the effects of things that other people have said to us about our appearance.

Our body image is also driven by our emotional state. You may have experienced big changes in how you feel about your appearance from one day to the next. Here's an example from Lauren:

*One day at yoga, I looked in the large mirror and I thought I looked absolutely fine. But the next time I was there, my emotional state was quite different. I'd had a bad day, and I'd fought with my partner, and when I looked*

*in the mirror, I thought I looked podgy and unhealthy. There were just a few days between sessions and of course my body hadn't changed dramatically in that short space of time. It was purely my emotional state influencing what I saw in the mirror. This highlights how subjective body image is.*

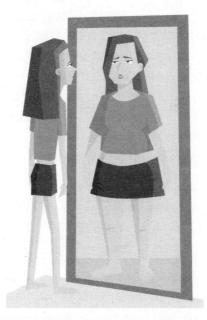

We are also driven by many assumptions about appearance: the idea that conventionally attractive people have an easier, happier, more successful life is prevalent in our society. The most attractive people feature in films and advertising campaigns, making us think that unless we're as attractive as them, our lives will be less fulfilling or successful.

Of course, appearance is important, and this book isn't about making you think otherwise. For example, we know that people make snap decisions based on appearance, and there is also a strong correlation between thinking that you look good and feeling good as a result. But there are a few things you need to keep in mind:

There are no universal laws on what constitutes an attractive person. Different cultures and different ages have prized all sorts of physical characteristics in men and women. For example, some elements of appearance that now seem to be absolutes used to be considered very differently. These days, thin is often sold as the ideal, but in many cultures and historically, curvy bodies were considered more attractive. Pale complexions were more highly prized than tanned complexions in the past, thin eyebrows were more fashionable than thick, and so on.

Appearance doesn't just refer to your physical looks. It covers the way you dress, your style, and how you wear your hair. It covers whether you wear accessories, adornments, body art or jewellery.

Above all, your appearance is not all you are. Neither is it responsible for all the bad things that happen in your life. So, while we don't dispute that appearance is important to you and the society we live in, your worth as a person is not dependent on how you look. Most people with body image issues believe that their appearance is the one and only indicator of their value. By the end of this book, we hope you will see that your physical appearance is only one aspect of you as a person. It's time to re-acquaint yourself with all the many, wonderful, unique, and precious things about you.

# BODY DISSATISFACTION, BODY IMAGE PROBLEMS AND BODY DYSMORPHIC DISORDER

The terms body dissatisfaction, negative body image, and body image problems are used to describe feelings of unhappiness with our body image. As we mentioned in our introduction in Part I, people who experience this kind of dissatisfaction will compare themselves unfavourably with others and experience low self-esteem as a result. Their appearance will be on their mind a lot of the time, sometimes to the point of obsession.

This sense of dissatisfaction can escalate into an obsessive preoccupation with any aspect of a person's appearance, including:

- Skin and complexion, including pores and skin tone
- Hair, particularly too much or too little hair on the head and body
- Size and shape of nose, ears, and mouth
- Body size and shape
- Asymmetrical features
- Other features such as moles, freckles, and scars

## BODY DYSMORPHIC DISORDER

Body Dysmorphic Disorder (BDD) is a diagnosable mental health problem in which a person obsessively worries about one or multiple flaws or perceived defects with their appearance. People with BDD believe they look ugly, unattractive, abnormal, or deformed. Other people do not notice these flaws or, if they do, see them as very minimal. People suffering from BDD carry out a number of repetitive and time-consuming behaviours or mental acts to try to hide the perceived flaw, or reduce the feelings of anxiety around it.

To be classified as BDD,[7] this preoccupation MUST cause serious problems in your daily functioning.

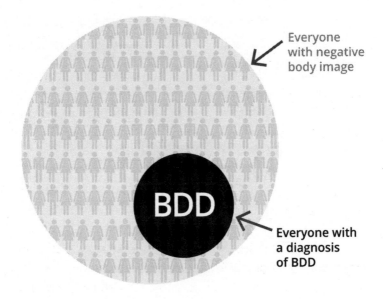

Everyone with negative body image

Everyone with a diagnosis of BDD

You can have negative body image without having BDD. However, everyone with BDD will have problems with negative body image.

If you are unsure whether you have a body image problem or whether you meet the criteria for BDD, don't worry, we'll help you find out. However, this book is for you, whether you have body image issues or BDD. The reason it can be helpful to know whether you have BDD as opposed to body image problems is that there may be additional treatment considerations for you. We'll discuss these as we work through Part II.

## MUSCLE DYSMORPHIA

Muscle dysmorphia is another form of BDD that mostly affects males. In this case, people believe that their body is too small, weak, or under-developed. In their efforts to deal with the negative feelings inspired by muscle dysmorphia, people often lift weights and exercise to excess. They may even take anabolic steroids or other substances to try to make their body bigger and more muscular. If you believe you suffer with Muscle Dysmorphia, then this treatment guide will help you too.[8]

## OTHER ASSOCIATED MENTAL HEALTH PROBLEMS

There are other mental disorders associated with poor body image and BDD, as well as co-morbid problems – mental health issues that you have alongside a body image problem or BDD. We have listed some of the more common ones here, but this list is not exhaustive and is just for guidance:

### EATING DISORDERS

Eating disorders include Anorexia Nervosa and Bulimia Nervosa, in which negative body image is part of the diagnosis. These disorders can be diagnosed alongside BDD. Anorexia Nervosa is where individuals restrict their food intake due to an intense fear of putting on weight, or becoming overweight. They generally carry out behaviours that interfere with weight gain, despite being underweight. Bulimia Nervosa is characterised by recurrent periods of binge eating, i.e. eating larger than normal portions in one go, a lack of control over eating, and behaviours to prevent weight gain such as vomiting, use of diuretics and laxatives, and excessive exercise. These eating disorders require specific treatment that is not covered in this book, so please do seek additional help from an appropriately trained therapist.[9]

## OBSESSIVE COMPULSIVE DISORDER (OCD)

OCD is another obsessive compulsive disorder like BDD. It manifests itself in unwanted intrusive thoughts, urges, or images ("obsessions") which are recurrent and persistent. These are combined with repetitive behaviours or mental acts ("compulsions") intended to deal with, or to avoid, such obsessions. For example, intrusive thoughts about becoming contaminated with bacteria may lead to time-consuming hygiene practices, including excessive handwashing and showering. OCD is also commonly diagnosed alongside BDD.[10]

## EXCORIATION (SKIN PICKING DISORDER)

This is an obsessive condition that makes a person feel compelled to pick their skin, resulting in skin lesions. Often this is in spite of their attempts to stop picking.[11]

## TRICHOTILLOMANIA (HAIR PULLING DISORDER)

Trichotillomania is an obsessive condition that makes people unable to resist the urge to pull out the hair from anywhere on their body, e.g. their head, eyebrows, eyelashes, or other areas, despite efforts to stop. The consequence is hair loss and this can cause significant impairment in a person's life in some way.[12]

## SOCIAL ANXIETY DISORDER (SOCIAL PHOBIA)

A fear of how someone will be scrutinised or judged in public. It can apply to any situation where they feel "on show" and at risk of being negatively judged by others. Sufferers avoid specific social situations or interacting with other people, or else they engage in safety behaviours when they are in their feared situation. For example, someone worrying that other people might find them boring or dull might drink too much alcohol at a party to feel more relaxed and confident, and to stop themselves worrying so much (but this in fact makes them worry more the next day because they can't clearly remember what they said or how they acted).[13]

## PANIC DISORDER

People experience panic attacks, which are feelings of sheer terror that strike suddenly with no warning and reach a peak within minutes. Panic attacks cause people to worry that they might lose control of themselves in some way or may be having a heart attack or mental breakdown. While panic attacks are common in all the anxiety and obsessive compulsive disorders, in Panic Disorder the sufferer fears having more panic attacks and goes to great lengths to avoid situations in which they worry they might have a panic attack. This can even leave some people housebound as they worry that as soon as they leave their house they may have a panic attack. Panic attacks are a result of heightened anxiety, and regularly occur among sufferers of any anxiety problem. It is the fear of having more panic attacks which gives the diagnosis of Panic Disorder.

## GENERALISED ANXIETY DISORDER (GAD)

People with GAD might sometimes be described as worriers. A bit harsh, perhaps, but GAD is defined by excessive and uncontrollable worry for reasonably long periods of time, and people find it difficult to control the worry. The worry can jump from subject to subject and can lead to worry about worry itself. People will also have physical symptoms such as restlessness, irritability, muscle tension and sleep problems.[14]

While this is not an exhaustive list of mental health problems, it covers some of the other obsessional problems, disorders that have body image problems as part of their diagnostic criteria, or ones that are more likely to occur alongside body image problems or BDD. If you believe you have one of these other problems instead of, or alongside, your body image concerns, it might be helpful to see a psychologist or psychiatrist for a diagnosis. However, if you suffer from body image problems or BDD even if you have another problem too, you will still benefit from reading this book.

What causes these problems? Well, we don't know exactly – as we have previously mentioned, it can be a combination of traumatic or upsetting events, responses to the environment, changes in brain chemistry, genetics, or early experiences in life. What we can say, however, is that it is not as a result of weakness or faults of character. People with BDD and body image problems are very often hard on themselves, blaming themselves for their problems. But is it not their fault. No one would opt to have body image problems or BDD as they are anxiety provoking and often disabling problems. However, what we can take responsibility for is overcoming these problems and reclaiming our lives from body image problems or BDD.

## OTHER FEATURES OF A BODY IMAGE PROBLEM

In Part I, we outlined the main attributes of a body image problem and BDD that we'll be helping you to change in this section. So let's just recap on the features that are usually present to some degree in body image problems and BDD:

- **Self-criticism** – having a relentlessly critical inner voice commenting negatively on everything a person does, including how they look.

- **The belief that appearance is everything** – believing that appearance is more important than everything else about themselves.

- **Safety behaviours** – these behaviours are designed to reduce the chance of a person's flaws being seen, or to protect other people from having to see their flaws. These include camouflaging, checking, researching "solutions", grooming, comparing yourself to others, cosmetic or dermatological procedures, etc.

- **Avoidance** – another type of safety behaviour where a person avoids certain situations, people, or relationships.

- **Compulsions or repetitive behaviours** – these are also safety behaviours, and are present in BDD. These are things that a person feels compelled to do in order to stop a threat (of being seen, or to protect others from seeing them).

- **Reassurance seeking** – asking others for reassurance that they look okay, or that their flaw is not noticeable.

- **Rumination** – going over and over past events in their head.

- **Worrying** – thinking too much about future events in a non-constructive way.

- **Selective Attention** – focusing on information that they perceive as a threat and using that information to reinforce their negative beliefs.

- **Self-focused Attention** – focusing on themselves, how they feel and what they are doing.

In the next chapter, we'll tell you more about the CBT approach we'll be taking to help you overcome your body image problems or BDD.

## YOUR RECOVERY STARTS HERE – SUMMARY

- Body image does not refer to how we actually look – it refers to the **subjective representation or felt impression** of how we think we look.

- Our body image is influenced by our beliefs about our appearance, our current emotional state, assumptions about appearance, how we feel when we look in the mirror, and other people's reactions to how we look.

- Appearance will always be important to people, but society's idea of beauty changes a lot over time. There are no universal laws on attractiveness: different generations and different cultures all have different paradigms.

- **Our appearance does not define us** and does not determine our worth.

- **Body dissatisfaction, negative body image and body image problems** are all terms used to describe unhappiness with body image. These involve people having distorted perceptions of their body or body shape, believing they are ugly or unattractive, feeling anxiety or shame about their body, or feeling awkward or uncomfortable about their body. **Body Dysmorphic Disorder is a diagnosable mental health problem** which causes a person to **worry obsessively** about one or more perceived or minor flaws in their appearance, and because of this worry they engage in **compulsive or repetitive behaviours.**

- There are other mental health disorders that require body image problems as part of the diagnosis, or can commonly occur alongside body image problems or BDD.

# SECTION 2

# COGNITIVE BEHAVIOURAL THERAPY

The techniques we'll be using to help you overcome your body image problems are based on **Cognitive Behavioural Therapy (CBT)**. CBT is the study of the relationship between the things that happen in our lives, how we interpret them, and what our emotional and behavioural responses are. When we can understand the link between these elements, we can start to understand why we get stuck in certain unhelpful patterns, both cognitively and behaviourally, and then find more helpful strategies for the future.[15]

**The main elements of CBT are:**

- **Cognition** – essentially what we think. This includes our beliefs, assumptions, biases, thoughts, as well as our emotions and feelings.
- **Emotions** – our feelings e.g. anxiety, fear, happiness, excitement, anger, frustration and shame.
- **Physiology** – the way our body reacts on a biological level.
- **Behaviour** – what we do physically or mentally, or in the case of avoidance, what we don't do.

CBT is the best treatment that we have for obsessional disorders and anxiety problems like body image issues and BDD for a number of reasons, in particular:

1. **Based on evidence** – CBT is evidence-based. This means it is tested in laboratory settings, and the treatment strategies are then tweaked and honed based on the data that is generated following the tests.[16]

2. **It's up to you** – It is a skills-based treatment that gives you the tools and techniques to get better and maintain recovery on your own. There are no secret techniques known only to therapists; this understanding is available to all!

3. **Easy to follow** – It is a structured step-by-step programme that allows you to progress through the stages as your own pace.

4. **Short term** – CBT is designed to be a short term treatment; it doesn't take years to get better! Hopefully you will start to see positive results in weeks, not years.

5. **No pain, no gain** – While we certainly don't mean that you need to suffer needlessly through this treatment guide, we will be asking you to do things that may feel uncomfortable and generate some anxiety (don't worry, we'll give you the tools to cope). If you don't feel uncomfortable, or it doesn't feel like you're being pushed, then you might need to push yourself a bit harder to confront your worries.

6. **Results** – Most importantly, the outcome is measurable by the goals you set yourself, so you can see if you're making progress, and you will know when you have completed the treatment.

## SETTING GOALS FOR TREATMENT

To begin with, take a moment to think about what you want to get out of this process. Having achievable goals can be very important in helping you reach your final destination: a life free from body dissatisfaction and worries about your appearance. In order to help you achieve this, we'll need to set some smaller goals for you along the way – this will give you a yardstick against which to measure your progress and it will help you recognise what recovery will look like for you.

Here's a useful question to help you set the right goals:

> **How is the problem you're suffering from interfering in your life?**

For example, Chloe's BDD interfered to the extent that she couldn't hold down a full-time job and she avoided going out in public. Other people with body image issues may avoid relationships or physical intimacy, feel like they have to wear clothes to help mask their perceived flaw, or try to avoid certain people and situations.

It may help you to think about the things that you would like to do but do not have the confidence to do, or used to do and no longer do, because of your body image problems. So let's start there. Think about how your body image problem or BDD is affecting your life and write it down in the box below:

These are the things I would like to do, but don't, because of my body image problems or BDD:

Now, let's think about your specific goals in a bit more detail. To help, we'll break them down into short, medium, and long-term goals. For example:

In the short term (when you've finished reading this book) you want to be able to go to the local shop to buy some milk without panicking and feeling like you have to put on concealing make-up or clothes to hide the area of your body that you worry about. Or you might want to be able to get changed in the changing rooms at the gym without awkwardly hiding behind a large towel or going to the toilet cubicle to get changed.

In the medium term (within the next six months) you might like to be able to wear certain clothes you've been avoiding, go to places like the beach, or be able to appear in photographs with your friends and family.

In the long term (at a point in the future that you're comfortable with), you might want to feel like you can go to unexpected social events, pop out whenever you feel like it, or have a relationship without even stopping to think about how you look or what you're wearing.

**MY GOALS ARE ... Short-term:**

**Medium-term:**

_____

_____

_____

_____

_____

**Long-term:**

_____

_____

_____

_____

_____

***Table 1:*** *My goals for treatment.*

Now you have set your goals, let's recap on the type of treatment programme you are undertaking.

# COGNITIVE BEHAVIOURAL THERAPY – SUMMARY

- **Cognitive Behavioural Therapy (CBT)** is the study of the relationship between events in our lives, how we interpret them, and our emotional and behavioural responses to them.
- CBT helps us understand why we get stuck in unhelpful thinking (cognitive) patterns and harmful behavioural patterns.
- **Cognition** refers to our beliefs, assumptions, thoughts, emotions, and feelings.
- **Behaviour** refers to what we do, or don't do, physically or mentally in response to our thoughts and feelings.
- CBT is an easy-to-follow, evidence-based, short-term treatment which is very effective in treating body image problems and BDD.
- CBT gives you tools and techniques to help you get better and maintain your recovery on your own, and the results are measurable.
- In order to undertake CBT effectively, you should set yourself achievable goals. You can break these larger goals down into smaller, more manageable ones – for the short, medium and long term.

# SECTION 3

# MY BODY IMAGE CONCERNS

Before we do anything else, let's find out what your body image problem looks like, i.e. what are the main behaviours and problem areas you face? To begin with, ask yourself these questions:

- Do you dislike some aspects of your physical appearance?
- Do you spend a lot of time thinking about the parts of your body you dislike?
- Is your appearance the most important aspect your sense of self-worth?
- Do you worry when you think about what other people think of your appearance?
- Do you fixate on the same negative thoughts about your appearance?
- Do you avoid doing things or going out because of your concerns about your appearance?
- Do you spend a lot of time every day "correcting" your appearance or trying to make yourself look perfect?

- Do you try to cover up your perceived flaws with concealers, make-up or clothes?
- Does the way you think about your appearance negatively affect the way you live your life?

If you answered yes to any or all of the questions, it suggests that you certainly have some body image issues, which obviously, you know, or you wouldn't be reading this book. So the next thing we need to do is help you discover whether you are suffering with body image issues or whether you might actually have BDD.

## DO YOU HAVE A BODY IMAGE PROBLEM OR BODY DYSMORPHIC DISORDER?

Take a look at these questions and answer yes or no to each one. Circle your answer and then calculate your score at the end of each section. Then you can add up your score to get an indication of whether you have body image problems or BDD.

**Thinking about your body image (preoccupation with appearance):**

1. Do you think about your area(s) of concern / your defect / your flaw(s) in your physical appearance a lot? **YES / NO**

2. Do you still think about it even if you try not to? **YES / NO**

**3.** Do you think about it more than 3 hours a day?
**YES / NO**

**4.** Is your appearance the most important thing about you? **YES / NO**

**Scoring:** ___ / 4    2 to 3 YES's = Body Image Problem
4 YES's = possible BDD

**Doing things about your body image concern (associated behaviour):**

**1.** Do you deliberately check your area(s) of concern in the mirror, a reflective surface, or by touch?
**YES / NO**

**2.** Do you do this outside of your usual routine and many times a day? **YES / NO**

**3.** Is it very difficult / impossible to stop even if you try to? **YES / NO**

**4.** When thinking of your routine regarding your appearance

  **a.** Is it inflexible? **YES / NO**

  **b.** Does it need to be done a certain way? **YES / NO**

  **c.** Does it need to be done with a certain outcome?
  **YES / NO**

**5.** Do you repeatedly ask other people (friends / partner / family) about your appearance? (or did you used to do this a lot?) **YES / NO**

**6.** Do you change your clothes often? **YES / NO**

**7.** Do you compare your appearance to that of other people and / or to yourself in the past? **YES / NO**

**Scoring:** ___ / 9    4 to 6 YES's = Body Image Problem
7 to 9 YES's = possible BDD

**Interference in your life (clinical significance):**

**1.** Does your thinking about your area(s) of concern currently cause you a lot of distress? **YES / NO**

**2.** Does it stop you from doing anything? **YES / NO**

**3.** Does it interfere with your relationship / stop you developing a relationship with someone? **YES / NO**

4. Does it affect your ability to work or concentrate? **YES / NO**

5. Does it currently interfere with your social life? **YES / NO**

**Scoring:** ___ / 5    1 to 2 YES's = Body Image Problem
3 to 5 YES's = possible BDD

As a further check, you can also add up your score for each of the three sections. Again, the score will indicate whether it is likely that you have body image problems or BDD:

**TOTALS:** ___ / 18    **7 to 12 YES's = Body Image Problem
13 to 18 YES's = possible BDD**

Please do bear in mind that while these questions are a good provisional screening method, we suggest you consult a health professional to confirm a diagnosis of BDD.

## WHAT'S THE DIFFERENCE,
## AND WHY IS IT IMPORTANT?

BDD is a recognised mental health disorder, for which the individual may be prescribed medication and require a more intense psychological treatment plan. BDD is likely to be more severe in its presentation than body dissatisfaction issues and it can consume many aspects of a person's life because of their severe **preoccupation** with their flaws or perceived flaws. People with BDD will be more preoccupied with their body image concerns, i.e. they will think about them a lot more during the day. It will be harder for them to ignore these thoughts or distract themselves from them.

People with BDD also have **compulsive and repetitive** behaviours and rituals. Remember, BDD is an obsessive compulsive disorder: people with BDD find that the compulsion to do something is so strong, they are unable to stop themselves doing it.

People experiencing body dissatisfaction will have more flexibility in the way they behave, meaning that they won't feel the same compulsion to do these things. Even if they carry out safety behaviours, they won't experience the same compulsive drive to do them that someone suffering with BDD will have. For example, when Chloe was compelled to wear her scarf, she couldn't not wear it, even in 35-degree Celsius heat (95 degrees Fahrenheit). She was compelled to cover her neck, one way or another. By contrast, someone experiencing feelings of body dissatisfaction about their neck might choose to wear a scarf if they have one available, but may be able to go without it in extreme heat, despite preferring to wear it.

In addition, the impact of their illness severely limits daily functioning for people suffering with BDD. Whereas people with negative body image might avoid some social interactions or specific situations, they may still be able to live a relatively normal life, including going to work, attending college, having relationships etc. People with BDD will struggle to achieve these things, or will do so under incredible duress. For example, Chloe struggled with college, and was only able to hold down a part time job for one day a week while feeling incredibly anxious and distressed before, during and after her working day.

The diagnosis of BDD is not always entirely straightforward. For example, Annemarie has worked with a woman who had visible stretch marks following pregnancy. She wouldn't go swimming or wear certain clothes, she avoided intimacy with her husband, and would only get changed in the dark. Although the stretch marks were noticeable to others, her level of preoccupation with them meant that she did have BDD: the impact on her life was very severe. In comparison, we have also spoken to women with the exact same issue who have had a completely different reaction. One woman felt like her stretch marks were a badge of honour – a symbol of the process of carrying and giving birth to her children. Her stretch marks did not stop her living her life in any way.

So, whether or not there is a noticeable problem isn't that important. We are not disputing whether or not there is a noticeable difference. Instead this is a problem about your level of preoccupation, and the way in which you respond to the flaw (imagined or real). In turn, this magnifies its importance to you and the extent to which you believe it is noticeable to others.

> Dealing with body image issues and BDD isn't about being right or wrong about your appearance, or disputing whether there is a noticeable difference or imperfection with your appearance. It is about the level of preoccupation you have with your appearance and the things you do, or don't do about it, and the impact these preoccupations or worries have on your life.

## THE BODY IMAGE CONTINUUM

It might be helpful to think of body image issues on a continuum. They can range from mild to severe. At the severe end we are likely to see people who will meet the criteria for BDD.

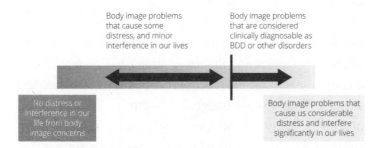

*Figure 2: Scale showing differing severity of anxiety interfering thoughts and behaviours.*

Regardless of how severe your problems are, we think everyone should be entitled to live a life free of these kinds of concerns. Even if you think your concerns are trivial but they still interfere with your life in some way, then it is still a worthwhile goal to strive to feel more comfortable in your body, and this book will help you.

Or, perhaps you are coming to this book believing you're living a very limited life due to your concerns around your body and appearance – like Chloe was – and you want to start being able to leave the house and meet people again. That is also an extremely worthy goal and it will help improve your quality of life significantly.

If you believe that you have BDD we also suggest that you might benefit from seeing your doctor and discussing all the available treatment options, including medication. But, don't worry, you can still follow this treatment programme and benefit from the tools and techniques we'll teach you in this book.

## MY BODY IMAGE CONCERNS – SUMMARY

- **Body Dysmorphic Disorder (BDD)** is a mental health disorder which causes a person to **obsess** about their body image concerns for a large proportion of the day and results in **compulsive and repetitive** behaviours and rituals.

- **BDD** has a **severe and often debilitating** effect on a person's life, causing them extreme distress and often preventing them from living their life or functioning normally.

- Body image issues are on a continuum, ranging from mild to severe. BDD would be at the severe end of the spectrum.

# SECTION 4

## STRESS, FEAR AND ANXIETY

As you read through this book, you'll see that we talk a lot about stress, panic, fear and anxiety. These terms refer to the same experience, and we all use the terms interchangeably. In fact, they are all referring to a normal human reaction to things that are perceived as threats. For ease, we predominantly use the term "anxiety" in this book when referring to this experience. Anxiety is an in-built, evolutionary alarm system that helps us respond quickly to threats. When we are faced with a threat, there are really only three choices – and they're the same choices humans have been making for tens of thousands of years: fight,

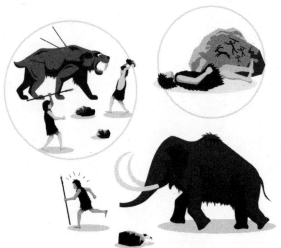

flight, or freeze. Whether you stand your ground and fight (fight), run away (flight) or hide and / or play dead (freeze), these are the actions that have helped keep humans safe for thousands of years.

So there's a sound basis for the fight, flight or freeze response. If your cavemen ancestors were being threatened by a sabre-toothed tiger, they needed to react quickly and they needed the extra surge of adrenaline to help them win their battle or outrun the tiger. Let's take a closer look at the effects:

What happens to the body when the fight, flight or freeze mechanism kicks in?

## Physiological effects of the fight, flight or freeze response

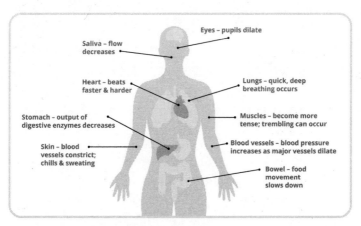

Eyes – pupils dilate

Saliva – flow decreases

Heart – beats faster & harder

Lungs – quick, deep breathing occurs

Stomach – output of digestive enzymes decreases

Muscles – become more tense; trembling can occur

Skin – blood vessels constrict; chills & sweating

Blood vessels – blood pressure increases as major vessels dilate

Bowel – food movement slows down

These are all the things your body does instinctively to make you stronger and faster and better when you face a life or death situation. But there's a problem …

## LIFE OR DEATH SITUATIONS?

No matter how scary it might seem to some people with body image issues or BDD, going to the beach with friends in summer isn't a life-threatening situation, or even a threat to your wellbeing. However, the strength of the fight, flight or freeze response still hits us just as hard.

As we've developed and evolved as humans, living in a fast-paced urban world, it gets harder to identify what a "threat" really is. Today's threats aren't just physical, they can be mental and emotional too. So while our threat system still operates just as strongly as it did for our ancestors, our threats are quite different. For example, the threat of losing your job could be just as anxiety-provoking, relatively speaking, as the sabre-toothed tiger was for the cavemen. Just because it isn't a mortal threat, it doesn't mean that the likelihood of losing income, incurring debt and struggling to provide for your family are any less terrifying in today's society. So for us, living in the twenty-first century, this is just as big a threat to our survival.

The things you do when you get anxious, (which are sensible responses to facing a sabre-toothed tiger) make a lot less sense when you're faced with social threats, such as the risk of rejection or humiliation. However, as we have pointed out, these are still threats to our survival in a socially connected, urban world. The difficulty is that our body is still responding in fight, flight or freeze mode, but the situation is often difficult to flee from. Imagine you are in a social situation, you feel very self-conscious, and you're worrying about your appearance. You could flee and go home, but that would be difficult to explain to other people, and in all likelihood, it will make you feel more self-conscious next time. You may feel frozen, which will make you feel more self-conscious, but it is unlikely you are going to start a fight! So the things that your body wants to do in those moments can often lead to worsening of the psychological symptoms – becoming more self-conscious and worried about what people think of you, which again is another threatening situation! So this is another vicious cycle in which the anxiety causes more anxiety!

So, we know that anxiety is a perfectly normal response, and we understand that everyone experiences it. (Yes, even those people we assume are always so confident and calm under pressure!) But it can be a big job for our internal appraisal system to manage these threats appropriately, and sometimes, we interpret events as much more threatening than they actually are in reality. Or we may believe that a threat is much more imminent

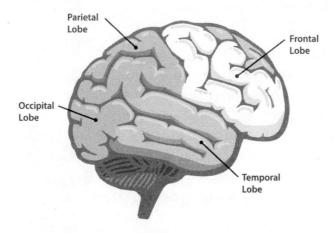

that it really is. This is an example of catastrophising – a thinking problem – that we'll tell you more about a little later. If you start thinking like this too often, then it is going to become a big problem.

In addition, in stressful situations the frontal lobes, which control reasoning, planning and problem solving, shut down because they're starved of oxygenated blood. So when our anxiety is high, our bodily response can make it difficult to think about things clearly and rationally – because our body is just trying to keep us safe!

## CALMING YOUR BODY DOWN

Sometimes it can be helpful to try different things that are physically incompatible with the physiological symptoms of anxiety. This can help our bodies calm down quicker and allow our brains to start processing again in a rational way. The quicker your anxiety tails off, the sooner the oxygenated blood flows back to the frontal lobes, helping you think more clearly.

Here are some more positive things you can try the next time you feel anxiety kicking in.

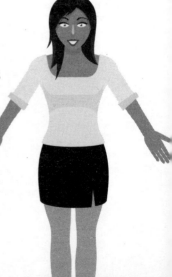

Using these kinds of strategies won't feel comfortable at first. Let's take the open body posture as an example. There's no point asking you to adopt an open posture when you're already in a stressful situation. You need to try it at home, on your own, in your bedroom. Practise getting more comfortable standing in a relaxed, open way. Don't huddle into your arms or fold them. Keep them relaxed by your side and lift your head up. Then, try it outside of your bedroom, and again when a friend comes round ... Keep doing it until it becomes comfortable, and then when you're in a situation where you feel anxious (but obviously there is no threat to your physical survival), it is easier to adopt an open posture. Over time, this sends your brain a different message and this means that your body will become less likely to respond in a fight / flight mode, making it easier to manage the situation.

It is remarkable what we can achieve by retraining our brain. Cognitively, behaviourally, and physiologically you can tell your brain to relax and ease off by adopting a different approach to your anxiety triggers.

## STRESS, FEAR AND ANXIETY – SUMMARY

- Anxiety is a perfectly **normal** human reaction to anything we perceive as a threat. When we perceive threats, we go into **fight, flight or freeze** mode. These responses are instinctual and have been with us for tens of thousands of years.

- The fight, flight or freeze response causes our bodies to quickly get ready for some kind of self-preservation action, so we experience a number of physiological symptoms.

- However, our living situations have changed since humans were cavemen and can now be harder to identify what a real threat is. **Threats can be mental (cognitive) and emotional too**.

- These kinds of threats or situations are not as immediately life threatening as, say, a sabre-toothed tiger, yet they are still threatening to our wellbeing in some way.

- We sometimes interpret situations as much more threatening than they really are, which will still cause us to experience the fight, flight or freeze response.

- You can calm your body down by trying different things that are physically incompatible with the physiological symptoms of anxiety – such as controlling your breathing, standing with an open posture, and keeping your head up, etc.

# SECTION 5

# COPING WITH DISTRESSING EMOTIONS

During your recovery journey, and as you work through these active treatment strategies, some things may trigger emotional distress. As we discussed in Chloe's story, people can find it difficult to cope with strong and overwhelming emotions and often avoid them altogether or find harmful ways of coping with them, e.g. through self-harm, substance or alcohol abuse. We understand these feelings are very unpleasant and difficult to tolerate, which is why you may want to avoid them or numb them. But there are other ways we can learn to get through these difficult feelings without having to avoid them or engage in unhelpful and often self-destructive behaviour.

If people use unhelpful ways of trying to get rid of emotions, they may come back in unintended ways. For example, if people self-harm and are caught out, they often feel embarrassed or ashamed about it, which then exacerbates the negative emotions. In addition, people who self-soothe with alcohol, drugs or sex with strangers might behave in an uninhibited way at the time, but find that when they reflect on it later, they're reminded of it, and feel more shame or embarrassment. So, the way people try to avoid these feelings can often make them feel worse in the long run.

We know that what you want to do, more than anything, is avoid feeling what you're currently feeling at that level of intensity. But, no matter what you do, you can't avoid the emotion. Whenever you avoid an emotion, it will just come back again. So, the most important thing to remember is that all feelings are impermanent. It doesn't matter which feeling it is – anxiety, depression, shame, loneliness, embarrassment, frustration etc. – even though it may be very intense and difficult to deal with, the feeling will not last at that intensity. In fact, if you monitor them over time, you will probably see that they fluctuate. Think about how you felt when you woke up this morning … Compare that with how you feel by the time you go to bed. Whether you feel better or worse, you're experiencing a different intensity of feeling. Maybe you're just in a different "head space".

### ALL FEELINGS ARE IMPERMANANT

It is a fact.

## IMPERMANENCE OF EMOTIONS

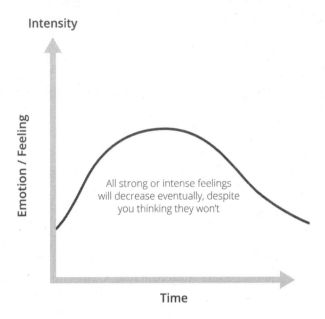

**Figure 3:** *Impermanence of emotions.*

So, no matter how unpleasant it is, or how intense it is, the emotion you're feeling is normal, and it will change and reduce. We know it feels overwhelming in the moment, but what you feel at the height of an emotional response will subside. And you need to ensure that you don't give it more strength – and make it last longer – by trying to avoid it.

## ACCEPTING YOUR FEELINGS

Accepting your feelings can feel very uncomfortable – counter-intuitive, even. Normally, when you encounter something so distressing, your first instinct is to try to "solve" the problem by hiding from it, or else avoiding it altogether. After all, that's what daily life teaches us. Think of all the advertisements you're bombarded with on a daily basis – if you have a physical pain, you fight it with painkillers. If you're unhappy with any aspect in your life, change it.

But actually, the more you try to avoid the feelings, or disguise them, the more the feelings will last.

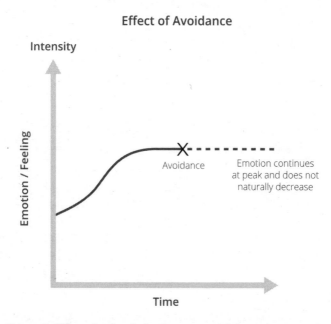

*Figure 4: Effect of safety behaviour or avoidance on our emotions.*

So, instead of trying to get rid of them, or "solve" them, you need to learn to cope with these emotions when they feel really strong.

Accept that you are feeling this way – don't judge yourself or the feeling. Remember that the feeling will not last. But what do you do while you're waiting for the feeling to reduce in intensity? We use what we call helpful distraction – focusing on activities that will help you get through this phase in a kind and compassionate way.

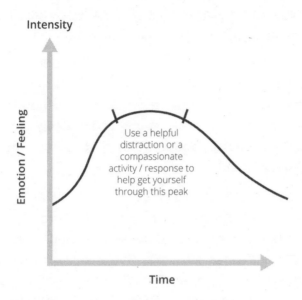

**Figure 5:** *How to manage strong emotions / feelings.*

## CHOOSE THE RIGHT KIND OF HELPFUL DISTRACTION

Helpful distraction means finding activities that will take your mind off the emotion. Everyone's preferred activities will be different – they may be slower paced or more active than others. What we want you to do is come up with a list of activities that will work for you. This could include going for a walk or a run, playing or listening to music, painting your nails, having a cup of tea, or even taking a shower – something that will help take your mind off your distressing feelings and focus on something else (and in so doing, stop you from focusing 100% on the difficult emotion). This will help bring your baseline stress level back to normal. There are hundreds of possibilities.

These activities are not a way of avoiding feelings; they show that you have made an active choice to do something, despite feeling bad, as opposed to doing something to try to not feel bad. Essentially, **you're acknowledging your unpleasant feelings and deciding to do something to get through them**.

A shower is a good example because there is that physical component to it. You feel the water running over you, you have to regulate the temperature, and these little things can help take your mind off the emotion. Or, think about taking a run at dawn. The cold air, the sun rising, the empty pavements – these things can really engage your senses and help your mind re-focus. Activities like these help you to be more mindful and pay full attention to the activity you're doing.

Make a list that will work, inside and out, day and night, at work and at home, so that whenever and wherever the unpleasant emotion occurs, you can deal with it in a constructive way. Here's an example:

## Take it easy
Do a crossword or sudoku
Arrange a hair appointment
Play a computer game
Read an inspiring book

## Get creative
Start a blog or journal
Join a class
Volunteer
Draw, paint or colour in
Sew or knit
Take some photographs

## Do something practical
Mow the lawn
Clean the car
Gardening
Cook something I love
De-clutter and
take things to
the charity shop

## Get out and about
Meet a friend
Go to the gym
Take it easy and watch TV
– without feeling guilty
Go and watch the clouds
Enjoy a gently stroll
somewhere nice

## Time to pamper!
Have an early night
Listen to some favourite music
Enjoy a nice, hot bath
Have a massage
Curl up with a drink and relax

## Write down your own helpful distraction techniques:

We acknowledge that, in the short term, drugs, alcohol, and self-harm might appear to give more of a kick, which helps to mask the unpleasant feelings, while the more compassionate strategies may not mask them completely. But actually, not masking your feelings is a good thing – because when you realise that you can tolerate your feelings instead of having to mask them, you will can stop resorting to self-destructive behaviours. You'll soon see that tolerating your feelings is the most compassionate thing you can do yourself.

## MINDFULNESS

We mentioned the importance of being mindful – in this context, we don't want you to judge or label the emotions you're feeling, but experience them and know them for what they are. It's about being in the moment.

Mindfulness is a very effective way of managing anxiety and worry and allowing thoughts or feelings into your head without judging them. Here is a brief mindfulness exercise for you to try:

1. Close your eyes
2. Take 10 or so deep breaths
3. Pretend you're somewhere that you find particularly relaxing
4. Try to clear your mind
5. As thoughts pop into your head, imagine turning them into clouds so you can watch them float off into the distance

Just remember that if you're feeling anxious and you can't stop thinking about it, then that feeling isn't going to subside because you keep fixating on it. You need to acknowledge that even while you're feeling anxious, you know it will pass. You also need to stop yourself from putting any negative judgement on it (e.g. it's awful, it's never going to end).

## REFOCUSING YOUR ATTENTION

Another useful tactic, which we'll also discuss when we talk about rumination, is choosing to actively shift your attention from an inward focus to an external focus. And we'll tell you how to do that in Section 11.

## OTHER WAYS TO STOP SELF-HARM

If you are trying to stop self-harming, a good technique is to make it physically impossible to do it in that moment. So if you cut yourself with nail scissors or a pair of tweezers, then try putting those things in a locked box and in a high up, hard-to-reach place. That way there is more of an obstacle to getting them, and people can see you reaching for it. Just stopping to pause and think can be enough to stop you from going through with it.

Similarly, if you physically depend on alcohol or drugs or prescription medications, making them more difficult to access or taking them out of the house altogether makes them harder to give in to. If it is more of an effort to go out and buy alcohol, it is likely to make you think twice about it.

A good example of this would be if, after a difficult break-up, you can't stop texting your ex after drinking.

To make it more difficult, you remove their number and any previous correspondence from your phone and don't store it anywhere. While this may not dampen the desire to do it, it does mean you'll be less likely to do it because it will be that much harder to do.

Another strategy might be to call a friend or family member to have a chat – you certainly don't have to tell them why you're calling if you don't want to, but it can be a good way to give yourself time for the feelings to reduce in intensity, and allow the desire to self-harm to pass.

It can be useful to make a list of alternative things you can do so when you experience the desire to self-harm, you can refer back to the list to remind yourself. Write down these things on the following page and put the list somewhere you can access quickly:

**Alternative actions:**

One of the key messages here is to learn to accept your feelings without avoiding them or trying to get rid of them. Remember that, no matter how uncomfortable your feelings are, they are **not permanent**. They will change at some point, maybe in a few minutes, maybe later on in the day. But they **will** change, and you **will** get through them; once you do, you can get back to working through this book.

## COPING WITH DISTRESSING EMOTIONS – SUMMARY

- Avoiding distressing emotions or using unhelpful behaviours to cope with difficult situations will lead to more distressing emotions, rather than fewer.

- No matter how unpleasant your emotions are, just remember that they are normal and that **they will pass**. They are always impermanent.

- You need to **accept** your emotional state rather than avoiding it or hiding it. There are other – more helpful – ways to deal with unpleasant emotions than simply avoiding them. A good way of managing them is to use **helpful distraction** – positive ways of distracting yourself in a compassionate way without masking the feeling completely or using harmful behaviours such as drinking or self-harm.

- **Mindfulness** and **Refocusing your attention** are also useful techniques which help you experience your emotions and accept them for what they are without judgement.

- A good way to try and stop self-harming is making it difficult to access the things that you would use to hurt yourself.

# SECTION 6

## IT'S ALL ABOUT HOW WE SEE THINGS

There are so many factors that shape the way we see the world – from the way we've been brought up, to the experiences that have shaped us – that no two people will see the world exactly the same.

### DIFFERENT TYPES OF THOUGHTS

It can be useful to think of these types of thoughts as different levels in a volcano, all pushing up so that the lava spews out at the top.

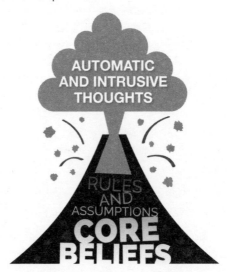

At the bottom of the volcano are the core beliefs – we don't see these as much – but they push through and influence our assumptions and beliefs, and in turn these influence the automatic thoughts we have. So in this example, the lava is the automatic or intrusive thoughts which are pushed out the top of the volcano by the pressure caused by our assumptions and rules.

Let's see how automatic thoughts work. For example, someone with body image issues or BDD may catch sight of themselves in a shop window and have the automatic thought: *That mole on my face is so big and ugly*. This comes from their assumption that they need to look perfect, or people will reject them. Sitting below this layer of thinking is the core belief that says appearance is everything.

Beliefs and assumptions are traditionally harder to challenge and change than automatic thoughts, as they are more entrenched and have developed over time. But the good news is that you are able to change them into more helpful beliefs and rules using the strategies in this book.

## EVERYTHING IS CONNECTED

To uncover your unhelpful thoughts and beliefs about appearance, we need to take a closer look at the relationship between what you think (your cognitions), how you feel (your emotional responses), how your body responds (physiology), and what you do physically or mentally (your behaviours).

Let's look at an example to demonstrate how all these things are connected:

Jonathan is called in to see his boss at work. He instinctively panics: *I made a mess of that job last week, I'm going to get fired*. And then his thoughts spiral out of control ... *I won't be able to keep up my mortgage payments. I'll lose the house. I'll be too embarrassed to spend time with friends ... How the hell will I ever find another job?* These worries make him feel so anxious that he makes an excuse, leaves work early and avoids the meeting. But this only helps to reinforce the likelihood in his mind that he is about to be fired.

But, if Jonathan thought about things differently, then he wouldn't need to leave work. So instead of fearing the worst (catastrophising), Jonathan thinks: *Okay, this is interesting ... I know I've been working hard. Maybe I'm going to get a promotion or some new responsibilities ... this could be a great opportunity*. As a result, he feels excited about the meeting and what it might mean; he tells his team that he'll take them for a drink after work.

In both cases, the situation is exactly the same, but the way Jonathan responds is very different in each case. He doesn't know what the meeting is about, and he can't predict the outcome of the meeting. But he can still choose how he thinks about the meeting, and then how he responds.

As you can see, our interpretations affect our emotions, physiological responses and behaviours.

That means that if we can learn to change our interpretations, we can change the way we feel, helping us to feel more positive and to respond in a more adaptive way.

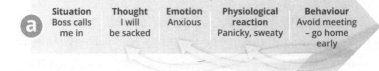

| | Situation | Thought | Emotion | Physiological reaction | Behaviour |
|---|---|---|---|---|---|
| **a** | Boss calls me in | I will be sacked | Anxious | Panicky, sweaty | Avoid meeting – go home early |

| | Situation | Thought | Emotion | Physiological reaction | Behaviour |
|---|---|---|---|---|---|
| **b** | Boss calls me in | I'm getting a pay rise! | Happy, excited | Jumpy from excitement | I'll buy the drinks! |

**Figure 6:** *How we interpret events affects our emotional, physiological and behavioural responses.*

Also, it is important to know that how we interpret an event or situation might be entirely different to how someone else interprets it. This is particularly relevant in the cases of body image problems, when we often feel very anxious because of how we have perceived things. For example:

Two friends are walking down the road, side-by-side. Someone they don't know approaches them, and as he walks past, he looks in their direction and laughs.

So how do they interpret that? One of them might think, *I wonder what that was all about ...* But then she lets the thought go, and forgets all about it. It was just a random event, so she doesn't have any strong emotional response. She just ignores it and keeps walking.

But the other friend has a different interpretation. To her, it counts as evidence that she looks weird or funny:

*Have I got something on my face? Does my hair look stupid? Did he think my clothes are terrible? I need to look in a mirror straightaway to see if everything's okay.* Even though she has no proof that the man even noticed her, the encounter makes her feel anxious enough to want to check her reflection as soon as possible.

This shows you how different people can interpret the same event in completely different ways, and that's why their emotional response, their physiological responses, and their resulting behaviours are completely different too. In one case, this chance encounter had the power to completely ruin someone's day, while in another case it was barely noticed and quickly forgotten.

So, what does this mean?

> **The way we interpret events affects how we feel and what we do in response.**

## THE WAY WE SEE THE WORLD IS INDIVIDUAL TO US

If you show a hundred people the same picture, they will react in a hundred different ways, based on their history, experiences and preferences. There is no right or wrong interpretation. Indeed, they can literally be seeing something different, because of the discrepancies in our biology which mean that we interpret visual information in different ways.

It is very hard to say whether what we're seeing fits with the reality of what we're looking at. Some time ago, an online debate about the colour of a dress escalated from a discussion on Facebook to an article in the *New York Times* and beyond! Everyone seemed to have an opinion as to whether the dress was blue and black, or white and gold. As people's perceptions were being called into question it left everyone who expressed an opinion feeling quite unsettled when their interpretation was called into question. Why? Because it can be destabilising finding out that other people see the same object in a very different way. We assume that our perception is accurate. We think the way we see the world is the way the world really is, but actually, the truth is less clear-cut.

## WHAT COLOUR IS A BANANA?

Let's take the way we experience colour as an example. The colour we see isn't actually in the object. The colour yellow is not in a banana skin; it's just that the surface of the banana reflects the yellow light wavelengths and absorbs the rest. The photoreceptors at the back of our eyes send the information about the light we're seeing to the brain, so that it can interpret it as colour. And because our photoreceptors will be stronger, weaker or arranged differently to one another, perception of colour will change a little or a lot from person to person.

So, no one else sees the world in quite the same way as we do, as individuals. The way people see and experience things depends on a combination of factors, ranging from past experience to the quality of light in a room. Everyone subconsciously brings their diverse range of experience to bear in interpreting everything they see and experience.

Do you remember that story about the doorbell ringing from Part I? It didn't take very long for Annemarie's beliefs to become really cemented in her head. That's because when we form an opinion and it turns into a belief, the belief is very hard to dislodge.

Here's another example of how that works. We met somebody who really disliked the 'bags under her eyes' – but it wasn't just because she thought they made her look older, it was because they reminded her of somebody in the family that she didn't like. So there was an uncomfortable association for her; without knowing it, she was cementing a negative belief. She also vividly remembered the comments people made about her eyes looking tired, which she attributed to the bags. So, her personal perception of this aspect of her appearance wasn't just affected by the image she had of herself in her mind's eye. Her feelings about somebody else, the comments about her looking tired and her emotional response to the comments all contributed to her dissatisfaction.

Everyone has imperfections – so why are we so bothered about ours?

As we've said – everyone has things about themselves that they would change if they could, and everyone has imperfections. So why do some people seem more anxious about them than others? Again, it is down to what we think it says about us and the value we put on appearance, i.e. our interpretation.

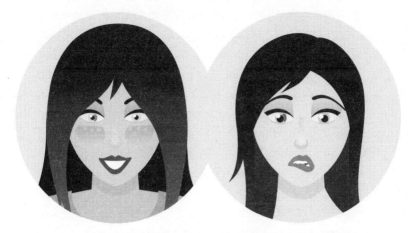

Two people with very similar characteristics can have very different interpretations of their physical characteristics.

One of our colleagues had a small, brownish patch in one of her irises which are otherwise blue. Her aunt and cousin have the same patch in their eyes, and she always liked having that connection with them when she was growing up. When she was at university, somebody noticed it, and said how nice and distinctive it was, which was a positive affirmation. Later, she met someone with a similar patch, of a different colour, who asked her if she was part of a support group. They explained it is a condition called heterochromia iridis. Our colleague didn't even know it had a name! What struck her was how the same feature could mean such different things to different people. To her, it was something she rarely thought about, but something that had positive associations. But for the person she met, it had more negative associations, and a greater impact on her day-to-day life.

So, the way we see the world, and ourselves, is unique. It affects how we feel, and consequently how our body responds, and then what we do, or don't do about it. In the case of body image problems or BDD, we view our body and appearance as one of the most important aspects about us, which then affects how we interpret other events and situations, such as how people look at us. This then affects how we feel emotionally, which causes us to behave in particular ways – known as our safety behaviours.

## IT'S ALL ABOUT THE WAY WE SEE THINGS – SUMMARY

- The way we **interpret** events or situations affects how we feel, how our bodies respond, and what we then do.
- Our **interpretations are unique** – no two people will see the world, or interpret things, in exactly the same way.
- People with body image problems and BDD see their body and appearance to be of utmost importance, which then affects how they interpret other situations and events.
- If we learn to change our interpretation of events, we can change the way we feel and react to situations.

# SECTION 7

# CAPTURING UNHELPFUL THOUGHTS AND IDENTIFYING THINKING PATTERNS

## CHANGING YOUR INTERPRETATIONS

So if the problem is due to the way we interpret events, or the way we see things, then we have to learn how to change this. Remember the example of the two friends walking down the street? One of them had interpreted the event as negative and believed the man they saw was laughing at her. So we need to identify what she was thinking and why that was unhelpful.

Before we can do this, we need to know what the situation is that triggers our unhelpful thoughts and responses. We call this the **trigger**. This is a situation, person, place – or anything that triggers your unhelpful thoughts and causes anxiety. It can even be anxiety itself. Intrusions are triggers too – these can be images, physical sensations, words and noises.

Take a moment to think about your triggers or trigger situations. If you can identify what they are, make a note of them here:

**My triggers:**

Your triggers might always be the same thing, e.g. getting changed in public spaces or going to the beach. Or they could vary, depending on the situation, the people around you, or how you feel. For example, some of Chloe's triggers were being in public without wearing her scarf or make-up, meeting people that were not her immediate family, using public transport, and having to talk to people she didn't know.

## CAPTURING UNHELPFUL THOUGHTS

The next step is learning how to catch the unhelpful thoughts in the first place. First you need to be aware of when you're having these experiences so that you can identify what the unhelpful thoughts and behaviours are.

Some people find it helpful to record when they're having these unhelpful thoughts. When you do this, you're looking for:

- The trigger

- The unhelpful thoughts

- How you feel and what you do (your safety behaviour)

There might be a difference, according to whether you have body image issues or BDD, in how these thoughts will manifest and whether you are aware of them. People suffering with BDD will probably be aware of their triggers, and they'll be very familiar with the kinds of thoughts they experience because the condition is constant and chronic. This extreme level of preoccupation often means they will experience these kinds of unhelpful thoughts all day! So it can be very time consuming to write down every single unhelpful thought. If this is the case for you, we recommend just noting down the most common thoughts and triggers – it will probably only be a handful of thoughts that repeat themselves.

Unhelpful thinking in someone with body image issues may occur less frequently and may not happen every day, so it's really important to capture those experiences when they do happen. Here's an example of how you can record the unhelpful thoughts:

Someone feels uncomfortable getting changed in a changing room at the swimming pool. After swimming, they think:

*Everyone is looking at me and noticing my wobbly thighs.*

They feel anxious and embarrassed and in response to these thoughts and feelings they keep their head down and get changed as quickly as possible, with a towel wrapped around them.

Let's look at another example:

> **The trigger:**
> I've been asked to go on holiday with my mates.
>
> **Thoughts:**
> Everyone is going to notice how thin and scrawny I am. It'll be embarrassing. I won't be able to enjoy the holiday, so what's the point in going and spending all that money? I feel sad and anxious thinking about it.
>
> **Behaviour:**
> I try to convince them to go somewhere a bit colder, so I won't have to take my top off, and I'm thinking of excuses of why I can't go with them if they decide to go somewhere hot.

If you find it hard to identify when you're having these thoughts, feelings of anxiety or distress will help you realise it's a good time to record what's going on. This will help you work out what you're thinking. Another clue is your behavioural response:

- Are you avoiding or planning to avoid something?
- Are you spending time on one of your safety behaviours?
- Are you ruminating?

If you find yourself doing these things, work backwards to help you identify the thoughts you were having, and the feelings you were experiencing.

A good way to help you understand what you're actually thinking is a technique we call "So what?" or "Why not?"

You will ask yourself questions at each stage of the process until you discover the true reason for the anxiety you're feeling. To illustrate this, here's an example about someone who doesn't want to give a presentation.

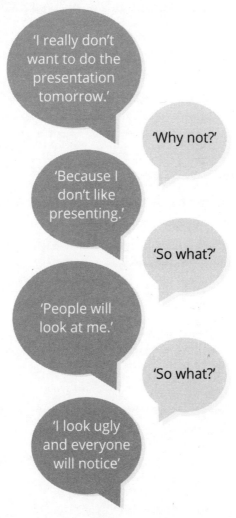

**Figure 7:** Example of "Why Not?" Or "So What?" questioning.

You can see that when he asks himself each question, he gets a little closer to identifying the core thinking at the centre of his anxiety. In this case, the employee worries that his peers think he's stupid and, by extension, is not fit to do his job. This thought may or may not be true, but it feels very real.

So, the next time you have an anxious feeling or an intrusive thought, try to work through this series of questions to find out what's at the bottom of it all. You might be surprised to learn what you're actually worried about! Try doing it in more than one situation to see if you're worrying about the same thing in all situations, or whether you have other core worries too.

You can follow the same format to record your triggers, thoughts and behaviours:

**What's the trigger event or situation?**




**What were your thoughts about yourself and your appearance?**

How did you feel?

_____

_____

_____

_____

How did you feel in your body?

_____

_____

_____

_____

What did you do?

_____

_____

_____

_____

**Table 2:** *Identifying my own thinking problems.*

# CAPTURING UNHELPFUL THOUGHTS AND IDENTIFYING THINKING PATTERNS – SUMMARY

- A trigger may be a situation, person, place, image, or something that triggers your unhelpful thoughts and anxiety.

- If you can spot when you're having unhelpful thoughts and capture the feelings and behaviours, you can identify the true reason for the anxiety you're feeling.

- When you get used to evaluating your intrusive thoughts, you might be surprised to discover what it is that you're actually worrying about.

# SECTION 8

# UNHELPFUL THINKING PROBLEMS

Once we have discovered our unhelpful thoughts, we can try to identity why they are so unhelpful (what we call thinking problems). These patterns of thoughts are "unhelpful thinking patterns".

These are some of the most common ones:

**WORST CASE SCENARIO or CATASTROPHISING**
Thinking the worst thing will happen in any scenario:
*If I leave the house without make-up, everyone will notice my bad skin, and think I look ugly.*

---

**PERSONALISING**
Thinking that everything is your fault or that it has something to do with you, even in cases when you couldn't have had anything to do with it, e.g. *They cancelled the work team photo – it must be because they don't want someone as horrible-looking as me in the photo.*

## BLACK AND WHITE THINKING or All OR NOTHING THINKING

Categorising things as good or bad, with no in-between: *I couldn't get out of the house today. I'm a failure. I'm never going to get past this.*

---

## CRYSTAL BALL THINKING / FORECASTING THE FUTURE

Thinking you can predict the future, or living as if the future has happened, e.g. *If I wear a swimsuit at the pool party next week everyone will notice how awful I look.*

---

## JUMPING TO CONCLUSIONS

Making a judgement, usually negative, even when there is little or no evidence for it, e.g. *Someone looked away as soon as they saw me; they think I'm hideous.*

---

## "SHOULD BE" and "OUGHT TO BE"

Thinking things HAVE to be a certain way, or people (including you) SHOULD behave in a particular way, e.g. *I should look better than this.*

---

## GUARANTEES ABOUT THE FUTURE

Needing everything to be guaranteed, or needing the outcome of events to be known, despite this being impossible, e.g. *I need to know that no one is going to stare at me before I go out.*

---

## EMOTIONAL REASONING

Basing things on how you feel, rather than reality, e.g. *I feel that I'm ugly, so therefore, I must be ugly.*

**PERCEIVED CONTROL or SUPERSTITIOUS THINKING**

Believing you have control over events or outcomes that you actually can't influence in any way, e.g. *If I check my appearance to make sure I'm looking professional before I make the presentation, it will all go well.'*

**OVERESTIMATION OF LIKELIHOOD OR PROBABILITY**

Believing an event to be imminent and inevitable, e.g. *There will be so many people in town and they will all be looking at me.*

**MIND READING**

Believing that you know what other people are thinking, despite having no evidence for it, e.g. *I know that everyone in this café thinks I look hideous.*

**DISCOUNTING POSITIVES**

Discounting any positive experiences so you only focus on the negative ones, e.g. *My boss said he liked the project, but that it needed to be devolved further, so he must actually have thought I hadn't really done a very good job.'*

**MINIMISING**

Downplaying the importance of something in an effort to make it feel, and seem, less significant, e.g. *My boyfriend said I looked beautiful, but I know he was only saying that to be nice.*

**SELF-CRITICAL**

Thoughts that are self-defeating and self-critical, e.g. *Why did I say that? It sounded stupid, now everyone thinks I'm a loser. I'm such an idiot for spilling that drink etc.*

**LABELLING**

An extreme form of self-criticism in which you give yourself a negative label, e.g. *I am useless, I am a failure, I am ugly.*

***Table 3:*** *Common thinking problems.*

This list is a careful selection of the many thinking problems people engage in, and we're sure there'll be some that you can identify with. For example, Chloe engaged in a number of thinking problems:

**Emotional reasoning:** She "felt" ugly, therefore that became her reality.

**Worst case scenario or Catastrophising:** Thinking the worst thing would happen if she went out.

**Mind reading:** Believing she knew what other people were thinking about her.

**Crystal ball thinking:** Believing she knew what was going to happen if she went outside.

**Labelling:** Believing she was "ugly" and "deformed".

Have a think about one of the trigger situations you wrote down in the last chapter, or a recent event that made you feel anxious and self-conscious about your appearance. What were your unhelpful thoughts? And what were the thinking problems you engaged in? What are the most common thinking problems that you seem to find yourself using? (It's all right if you say it's all of them!)

Don't worry if more than one thinking problem seems to fit. It's not a perfect science and more than one type of thinking problem can apply to a single thought.

**My most common thinking problems ...**

*Table 4: My most common thinking problems.*

## THE UNHELPFUL CYCLE OF ANXIETY

We have seen how easy it is for an unhelpful cycle of thinking and worrying to begin, and once it's begun, it can be very hard for people to get out of it again. What makes it harder is that all the various elements interact with each other, helping to reinforce the anxiety.

If you have body image issues or BDD, you will interpret an event in an unhelpful way and will engage in at least one thinking problem. Your emotional responses are likely to include anxiety, fear, worry, doubt and panic. Your body will feel on "high alert" as it goes into fight, flight or freeze mode. As a result, your behaviour – which is intended to reduce the feelings of threat and anxiety – will be safety-seeking behaviour or avoidance. And, as we have seen, that will only reinforce your anxiety.

Here's an example to show you how that works if you are scared of going to the dentist:

- Your trigger is the thought about going to the dentist.
- Your interpretation is that it will be painful and you will not cope with the anxiety.
- Your body feels sweaty and hot.
- Your behaviour is avoidance.

In avoiding going to the dentist your body feels sweaty and hot when you think about it, and so you avoid going to the dentist entirely. But in avoiding going to the dentist, your belief that it will be painful and you won't be able to cope can't be disproved. Therefore, avoiding the dentist also reinforces your belief and your fear – and it means you remain locked in this cycle of anxiety and it will re-occur every time you think about the dentist.

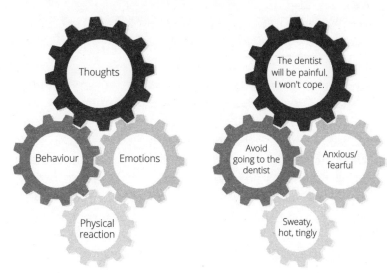

**Figures 8 & 9:** *The interaction of our thoughts, emotions, behaviours and physiological reactions.*

Even worse, if you have a toothache and you avoid the dentist, the physiological consequence is that the toothache will only get worse; it may even require more serious treatment at a later stage. In Part I, we discussed an example of someone who might wear a hat to hide a bald spot, or sunglasses to hide bags under their eyes. Both would both have the unintended consequence of drawing more attention to appearance.

In this case, we can see that one of the **unintended consequences** of this behaviour is an untreated tooth. So we can see that avoidance itself can make the problem worse in many ways!

# IT'S TIME TO CHANGE THE WAY YOU THINK ABOUT BODY IMAGE

Once you're aware of your triggers, thoughts and thinking problems, you can start to change your interpretation of your body image.

As we said, people assume that how they see the world is how everyone else sees the world. So they inevitably think that their reality is fact. Therefore, if you have a negative body image, you will assume that everyone sees the exact same imperfections that you do. But of course, other people's realities will be very different to your own. Hopefully by now you are starting to get used to the idea that what **you** see is different to what **others** see. Then, as a result, you can change those unhelpful thoughts to thoughts that are more realistic and helpful.

You are going to learn to consider different perspectives or interpretations of events about any given situation. For example, imagine you're out walking and you see somebody looking in your direction. Your instinctive belief might be, *They think I'm ugly*. This is clearly a **mind reading** thinking problem. One alternative explanation is that they like your outfit. You might feel inclined to discount that possibility straightaway. But we would ask you to accept that you cannot actually know what they were looking at. Nor can you say with any certainty that they were looking because they thought you were hideous. We cannot say that your interpretation is absolutely wrong; we accept it as a possibility. All we're asking is that you accept that another interpretation is possible, even if it is something you have not considered, or it is something you have actively discounted.

Let's think about some questions that will start to change the way you think about your body image:

1. Is this thought helpful? It would be considered unhelpful if it makes you feel distressed or anxious after having the thought, and if it makes you engage in a safety behaviour or avoidance.


2. Is it 100% true, i.e. do you know it for fact? (That is different from **feeling** that it is true; that would be a thinking problem called **emotional reasoning.**)


**If the answer to either of these questions is no then ask yourself:**

3. Is there one or more thinking problem at work here? See the beginning of this section for a list of the most common thinking problems.

**4.** What is the evidence for this thought?

**5.** What is the evidence against it?

**6.** What could be a more helpful way to think about this? Even if you don't think the new thought is likely?

**7.** If one of these alternative interpretations was true, what difference would it make to how you feel?

**8.** If one of these alternative interpretations was true, what difference would that make to the action you would take?

## CHALLENGING YOUR
## UNHELPFUL THOUGHTS

You will need to practise challenging your unhelpful thoughts like this. To begin with, it can be difficult to do in the moment when you're feeling especially anxious, so you might have to think about it after the trigger event. Let's say someone pushes past you at a party. You might immediately assume that it happened because they wanted to get away from you as quickly as possible. At the time, when you are stuck in those terrible feelings of anxiety, it can be really difficult to think about it differently. But afterwards, once your anxiety reduces you can consider some of the other possible reasons. For example:

Maybe they were just clumsy. Or they were rude and thoughtless, and that's why they didn't apologise. Or maybe they were in a hurry for some reason and couldn't stop to say sorry.

As you get more practised at doing this, you will be able to do it as these events happen. Once you have a new way of thinking about events, you'll be able to apply it quickly in situations, and it will start to feel normal to do so. This new way of thinking will also help you respond in different ways, so instead of engaging in a safety behaviour or avoidance, you can choose how to respond in a more helpful way.

## THE TWO HANDS THINKING TECHNIQUE

We know that living with BDD or body image issues is hard work. We appreciate that all of the things you've tried to make things better haven't worked. That is because in all probability, as we have indicated, the problem isn't your appearance; the problem is your worries about your appearance.

With any body image or BDD-related issue, there are two hypotheses on what the problem is:

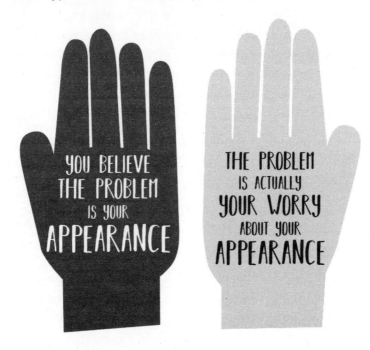

**On the one hand, you believe the problem is your APPEARANCE.**

**But on the other hand, the problem is actually your WORRY about your appearance.**

We call this the Two Hands Thinking Technique – and you are going to use it to help change the way you think about your body and your appearance.

Here are a couple of examples:

Meet Adrienne. She believes that her nose is too big. In fact, she hates her nose. And that train of thought leads her to believe that her boyfriend will find someone "more attractive" and will eventually break up with her, meaning she'll be alone for ever.

As a result, Adrienne might consider surgery, or she might try to minimise the size of her nose with clever make-up. She doesn't want people seeing her from a certain angle, so she might try to sit in such a way that people only see her 'good' profile. She might even try to reduce her social contact altogether. She would probably also spend time researching 'normal' noses, so that she can gauge how 'bad' hers is in comparison to others. Adrienne has developed certain behaviours designed to minimise the look of her nose, or to stop other people from looking at her. These will fall into different categories:

- Checking or monitoring her image – by touching her nose, looking in the mirror, or thinking about how she feels.
- Camouflaging – using clever make-up and shading to minimise the appearance of her nose.
- Comparing – comparing her nose to other people's noses (including photos she sees on Instagram and Google).
- Avoiding – this includes minimising social contact and avoiding certain lighting conditions.
- Other safety seeking behaviours – e.g. only showing her profile, looking at cosmetic surgery options, saving up for cosmetic surgery.

- Ruminating – going over and over the worries in her head, or the experiences she has found embarrassing or anxiety-inducing.
- Reassurance seeking – asking her boyfriend and her family if her nose looks weird or if it is too big.

These are the solutions (or as we know them, safety behaviours) that she has been relying on for several years. She believes that they are necessary in order to live her life as normally as she can, despite the obvious interference.

Let's look at Adriene's problem using the Two Hands Thinking Technique:

**On the one hand ...**

Adrienne believes 100% that the problem is her appearance. She "knows" that if her nose was smaller or more attractive, her life would be easier.

This is a hard belief to shake. Not least because if it is noticeable to her, then she thinks it must be just as noticeable to everyone else.

**On the other hand ...**

The problem is one of Adrienne **worrying** about the size of her nose. So really it is a worry problem, not an appearance problem.

Adrienne's problem is actually her body image – in other words, the feelings and felt impressions that she has relating to her appearance. The problem we need to address is not her nose; it is her worry about her nose, and her preoccupation with it. If you treat it as an appearance problem when it is a worry problem, you won't address the real issue. That would be like treating a person for cancer when they only have a deep-rooted fear of cancer symptoms.

The other issue is that Adrienne is living her life as if her problem is actually her appearance, not that the problem is one of worry. As a result, all her safety behaviours and avoidance are because she believes that her appearance is the problem and that she needs to do these things in order to make the size of her nose less of a problem. However, the reason people engage in safety behaviours and avoidance is because of their anxiety, not because of a problem with their appearance. Think about it: does the process of checking and monitoring make you less anxious or more anxious? Most people can see that actually, it makes their anxiety worse. Not convinced? Let's put it to the test then.

Imagine that your exam results are coming in between 9.00am and 11.00am. Now, on the one hand, you could check your email account 300 times from 9.00am, trying to get your results as soon as they become available. But they don't actually come in until 11.05am. You rate your anxiety before and after checking every time and see that your anxiety is spiking on every occasion.

In a different version, you make a conscious decision to just get on with life and log in to check later. You check your email shortly after 11.00am and get your results.

In which version are you more or less anxious? Why?

Of course the first version would make you more anxious. That process of repeated checking actually elevates anxiety. So, if the problem is a worry problem – not one of appearance – then all that checking and monitoring is going to make the anxiety and worries worse!

What about avoidance? Well, we know that fear and avoidance have a best-friend relationship. If we are worried about something and we avoid it, our fear of it goes up. For example, if you're at work and your boss asks if he can have a word with you, you might immediately think 'Uh oh, I've done something wrong' and feel anxious. Then the phone rings – it gives you an opportunity to avoid the meeting with your boss: 'Oh, sorry, let me just get this ...' At the time, you feel this nice sense of relief flood over you, but then, the next time you see him come out of his office, the fear flares up again. When you avoid something that makes you anxious, the relief you feel is fleeting, and kicks in again as soon as a trigger activates it again. So you can see that avoidance is further evidence that you have a worry problem.

Now, we know it might be difficult to accept that your issue isn't an appearance issue. But we've got two hypotheses on what the problem is, so let's find out which one fits so we can find the best solution.

Let's take a closer look at the two options using an example from Chloe's experience:

**On the one hand my problem is ...**
The problem is that my neck sticks out. It looks hideous. Everyone will notice and be repulsed.

**How am I living my life because of this:** (i.e. what am I doing to make sure my fears do not come true and to reduce my anxiety?)

- I am covering up my neck.
- Avoiding seeing my friends, avoiding going out.
- Avoiding certain types of clothes.
- Checking my appearance / neck in the mirror or any reflective
surface and comparing myself to others
- Not going to school.
- Evidence for this position being true?
- I think my neck looks weird.

**On the other hand ...**

The problem is that I am **worrying** too much about my neck and **worrying** too much what other people think of me / my appearance.

**Ways I could live my life if this was only a worry problem rather than it being real:**

- I wouldn't have to spend hours doing all my safety behaviours
- I could live my life how I want to live it
- I would focus instead on building up my confidence, and most importantly, I could stop worrying so much.

**Evidence for this position being true:**

- No one has stopped me in the street to comment on my neck
- Nobody has said anything to me about it at school
- No medical professionals have ever said it was abnormal
- I worry about other aspects of my appearance, so it's likely that I would worry about other things too

> - I was never teased about my neck
> - I have an identical twin sister and I can't see any problems with her neck

**Table 6:** *An example of a completed form showing On the One Hand vs. On the Other Hand.*

Having read Chloe's story, which of the **"Two Hands"** explanations do you think is actually true for her?

> **Of course, Chloe's problem wasn't that her neck was deformed and would offend people; her problem was that she WORRIED that her neck looked deformed, and she WORRIED about shocking and offending people.**

This might seem like an easy conclusion to reach, but it really wasn't for Chloe. She was absolutely convinced she was so disfigured that people would be shocked and repulsed by her. Based on that belief, that she went to some extreme lengths to avoid subjecting herself to that kind of public scrutiny.

To help her decide which of the "Two Hands" explanations was true, we encouraged her to **weigh up the evidence** for herself. Had anyone ever reacted with such shock or revulsion in her presence? Had anyone made fun of her because of the way her neck looked? Had any medical professionals ever spoken to her about what was such an obvious problem? Had any of the therapists and counsellors she'd met ever agreed with her that there was an obvious problem? Did she have any more objective evidence for her belief?

The answer to every one of these questions was "NO". There was no evidence that Chloe was a "gargoyle" as she described herself. There was no evidence to suggest that people would have been offended or shocked by her appearance.

Again, if it's true that Chloe's problem was one of worrying about her appearance and what people thought of her, how could she live her life differently?

Well, for a start, she could leave her house when she wanted, and wear what she wanted. She could work on her career and travel to see friends. We know these things might be hard to imagine, but if your problem is one of worry, then you are beginning to see how your safety behaviours and avoidance are actually reinforcing the idea that the other position is true – that it is your appearance that is the problem.

> **If your problem is one of worry, then your safety behaviours will never help you.**

## BEGINNING TO SEE THINGS ANOTHER WAY

- You can see that changing how you think about your appearance is key to changing how you feel and your behaviours.
- You can do this by identifying trigger situations and identifying whether your thinking is helpful or accurate, and then working out what your thinking problems are, before coming up with another more helpful way of thinking.

- You can use the **Two Hands Thinking Technique** to help challenge your beliefs about your appearance.

- Weighing up evidence using the Two Hands Thinking Technique helps you see which interpretation of the problem is more likely.

- You will be able to see that the problem is one of WORRYING about your appearance, not actually a problem about the way you look. Therefore, you can start to live your life free from the rigorous and demanding safety behaviours, and free from avoidance.

And yet, despite all of this learning, you still feel bad ... Of course you do! We know that body image issues, BDD and the anxiety they bring don't give up quite so easily. You may have discovered their nasty little secret, but that doesn't mean they'll just slink away.

But don't worry. Now that we have a new way of understanding that the problem is actually a worry problem about your appearance, we can start to modify your behaviour to match. Over the next two chapters we will help you find the confidence you need to drop your old safety behaviour methods, and start testing out this new way of thinking about your problems.

# UNHELPFUL THINKING PROBLEMS – SUMMARY

- Thinking problems are patterns of unhelpful thoughts. If you think about one of your trigger situations, you can identify your thinking problems – there may be one or many.

- If you interpret an event in an unhelpful way, your emotional responses will include anxiety, fear, worry, doubt and panic.

- You can change the way you think about experiences and situations, including how you think about your body, appearance and other people.

- The Two Hands Technique is one helpful strategy to challenge old unhelpful ways of thinking.

- It is likely that the problem is actually your worry about your appearance.

# SECTION 9

# TESTING IT ALL OUT

Now that you've got used to the idea that there is another interpretation of the body image problem you've been living with, we'll talk you through some useful experiments to test out your new interpretation of your problem, and help you face the fearful situations.

## FACE THE FEARS?!

That's right. To help you overcome body image issues and BDD you need to go right towards the feared situations and ... face them. It sounds weird, but actually, the more you do it, the easier it will be to get used to the things that are causing your anxiety. This is called habituation – and it's the best way of helping people get used to the things that scare them. By doing the experiments, you will get to the point where your trigger situations or events no longer provoke fear.

Now, bear with us here. We do know that what we're asking you to do runs counter to normal instincts for combating your anxiety problem. So far, you've run away from the issue, or pushed it aside with your safety behaviours, or avoidance strategies. And maybe that has even helped you feel a bit better – for a little while. But it hasn't taken the problem away – or else you wouldn't be reading this now. If anything, it's probably made the problem more entrenched.

So, it's natural for you to have doubts. We've yet to meet anyone in therapy with body image problems and BDD who doesn't have doubts about the process we're going to follow, especially when it comes to embracing their issues. 'There's no way I can do THAT!' people tell us. If you remember, Chloe couldn't even think about moving her scarf from around her neck to begin with.

The likelihood is that you've lived so long with body image issues that you're bound to feel nervous as we go into this stage of the programme. But please stay with us; these methods work.

## SO WHAT IS HABITUATION AND HOW DOES IT WORK?

Habituation is a process that happens when we expose ourselves to previously avoided or feared situations. At its simplest, this is a way of helping you get used to something that used to scare or upset you. It's based on the very simple theory that the more you do something, or the more you are exposed to something that you find unpleasant, the more you will get used to it.

This applies in other ways too. When you hear a favourite song on the radio, your ears will prick up and you'll listen intently. But if the song gets played every day, you'll get used to hearing it. You have habituated to the sound and barely notice it any more.

You can use this technique to help you habituate to the things you don't like so that they stop bothering you so much. For example, if you are afraid of spiders, you can try things that will gradually help you get more used to seeing spiders. This could start with looking at pictures of spiders in a book and culminate with going to the arachnid house at the zoo, and perhaps even holding one. You may never get to a point where you particularly like spiders, but if you've been living with a mortal terror of seeing them crawl across the floor, you will really feel a positive difference.

The key thing with habituation experiments is that you do them without resorting to your old safety behaviours. Imagine you're about to dive off the highest diving board you've ever seen. It's a terrifying prospect, but you manage to jump. And then you do it again, and again ...

By the fifteenth time, it doesn't feel terrifying any more. That's because you have habituated yourself to the experience. But if you had resorted to a safety behaviour every time, e.g. closing your eyes for the jump, or even avoiding it altogether, you would still be terrified by the prospect of the fifteenth jump (or any jump if you chose to avoid it entirely).

Take a look at the graphs. The first one shows what happens when you come up against your trigger and you make your anxiety go away using your tried and tested avoidance and safety behaviours:

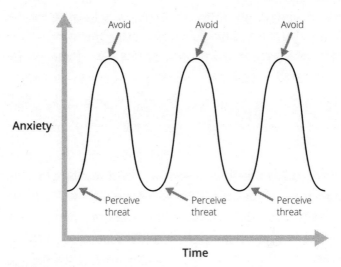

**Figure 10:** *Avoidance of threat.*

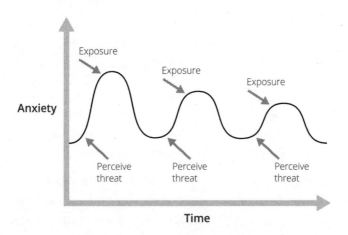

**Figure 11:** *Exposure to threat / habituation of anxiety.*

Every time you detect a threat, your anxiety level shoots up until you carry out a safety behaviour and it drops back down again, but only temporarily. Because the next time your anxiety is triggered, it shoots back up again until you perform your safety behaviour and bring the anxiety back down. And on and on it goes. Nothing ever changes. And nothing is ever done to reduce the anxiety permanently.

In the second graph, you can see what happens when, instead of avoiding your trigger, you expose yourself to it and face it:

Here you can see that, if you face the threat by exposing yourself to it, the level of anxiety you feel will actually decrease over time. Like in the example above, let's say you have a phobia about spiders, and your anxiety shoots up when you see one. So obviously, under normal circumstances you'd try to avoid spiders whenever possible so you don't have to subject yourself to that fear. But then, the next time a spider runs across the floor, your anxiety spikes again. So avoiding the trigger clearly didn't make it any easier to deal with a spider the next time you encountered one.

So, here's a scary prospect ... Instead of encouraging you to try to avoid spiders, let's say we're coming to meet you, and we're bringing a spider in a box with us!

Now, instead of avoiding the situation, you stay in the room with the spider. You're obviously going to feel very uncomfortable in that situation, but, if we bring a spider with us every time we come to meet you, we guarantee you will start to feel a little less uncomfortable. Instead of retreating from the thing that makes your anxiety spike, you are habituating yourself to it. And the longer it goes on, the faster your anxiety will reduce. Your brain will learn that the threat is not actually as bad as you'd feared, and your body will respond accordingly. You'll start to feel calmer and more assured.

Because the perceived threat of the spider has not resulted in any actual danger, your body can't help but respond to that fact.

You survived the first time. Maybe it was just a fluke. You survived a second time. Lucky again? Third, fourth and fifth times … There's a pattern emerging. Maybe your feared outcomes weren't that likely after all.

Now, you might reasonably say that you're not going to go anywhere near the spider in the first place, let alone be in the same room as it. And we can absolutely understand that reaction. Whatever your trigger is, the anxiety around it has been working its way into your head for so long that it's inevitably going to feel very strange to confront it, head-on, and see it for what it is.

Let's use a story to help describe this part of the process:

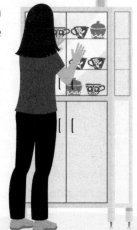

An antique dealer employs an apprentice. When he walks the apprentice onto the shop floor, the apprentice notices a heavy sweeping brush propped up against the door of a cabinet. The door is made of glass, and behind it the apprentice can see lots of antique glass bowls and plates stacked on the shelves. The antique dealer tells the apprentice that she needs to keep the cabinet door shut while he sweeps the back room with the brush, otherwise the bowls and plates will come tumbling out and smash onto the floor. The antique dealer takes the sweeping brush and goes into the back room and leaves her alone on the shop floor, unable to take her hands off the cabinet door.

Just then, a customer walks into the shop and asks her to serve him. By this time, the apprentice has been holding the door shut for a long time. But she looks worried and tells the customer she can't move until the antique dealer comes back. He asks her why.

'Because those glass bowls and plates are antique and very valuable. If I move my hand away from the door, the glass bowls will fall out.'

'What makes you think that?' the customer asks her, puzzled.

'Because the antique dealer said so,' replies the apprentice.

Instead of getting impatient and leaving the shop, the customer suggests that the apprentice moves her hand away from the door slightly. This worries the apprentice, but after thinking about it carefully, she decides to try taking her hand away from the door just by a couple of centimetres or so. She knows she will have enough time to stop the bowls falling out if she senses them starting to fall. As she moves her hand away slightly, nothing moves.

'Looks okay so far. Why don't you move your hand away from the door completely?' the customer asks.

'No, I can't do that. If I do that, they will all fall out and I won't be able to catch them when they do.'

'On the other hand,' the customer reasons, 'that might not happen at all. It might just be that you're worried this will happen. Why not give it a try?'

The apprentice, feeling nervous, moves her hand away completely and drops her hand down by her side. Again, nothing moves or falls out of the cabinet. The apprentice breathes a sigh of relief.

'Now, why not try opening the cabinet door?' the customer asks her.

The apprentice looks very worried about this. But the bowls haven't fallen so far, so she slowly and tentatively starts to open the door. Surprise, surprise – nothing falls!

The lesson is that you never know until you try, and it's just the same with your BDD or body image problems, and the anxiety you experience. Your safety behaviours are like holding that door shut. You don't actually know what will happen once you move your hands and open the door, but we all know that by holding it shut you're completely stuck. It may take courage, but once you can take that step (whether it's going out with a little less concealing make-up, or sitting next to someone on a bus) you will feel anxious but you will also learn whether or not you should be anxious in the first place!

## EXPERIMENTS

So what we're going to ask you to do is conduct a series of experiments around your concerns. For example, you might leave the house without one of your emergency hair products, or your hair straighteners, or without the hat that you normally use to hide your ears – or whatever it is that will challenge you.

You don't have to do this completely alone. Tell a friend or a relative what you're going to do. Perhaps you can arrange to discuss it with them afterwards. Or, if you're seeing a therapist, a CBT specialist, or a doctor, you might want to incorporate this exercise en route to seeing them, so you can review your progress afterwards. Sharing it as soon as possible **after the event** is a useful way to update your beliefs with the new information you learn from the experiment.

Now, take a look at these boxes. The first one gives you an example of an experiment, and the second one is blank for you to fill in with whatever experiment you choose. This isn't an experiment to push you to your limits and see how you react, it's to test if what you fear is really true.

To start with, you'll need to write down exactly what you intend to do in your experiment. Think about how you might feel before you start, and write down what the 'one hand' is telling you what might happen. Be honest! Here's an example of what that will look like:

---

**My experiment is to ...**
• Get on a bus to town without wearing any make-up


**On the one hand I feel ...**
• Nervous, anxious, sick

---

**And my worry says ...**
- That people will stare at me and move away from me because I am so ugly

**On the other hand ...**
My worry problem is telling me that I am WORRYING about what people will think and I will be anxious and feel really uncomfortable. But people are not likely to point or stare, or perhaps even notice me.

**Table 7:** *Example of setting an experiment.*

So what about you? What experiment will you try? For example, if you're afraid of going out in public without wearing a hat or some other concealing clothing, you can start by stepping outside your door for just five minutes and walking to the garage, the end of the driveway, or the end of the road. You don't have to speak to anyone, and you don't have to go anywhere else. Five minutes might seem like a long time at first, but we recommend that as a minimum because you need to be able to experience the anxiety, to see what happens next.

In Chloe's case, she planned to walk to the train station and back home without wearing her scarf. On the way back, she was going to stop for coffee. On the one hand, she was afraid that somebody was going to stare at her, or say something to her about her neck, or that they'd refuse to give her eye contact when she was ordering a drink. In response, she worried that she would feel so distressed that she wouldn't be able to speak. She also worried she'd

**My experiment is to:**

**On the one hand I feel ...**

**And my worry says ...**

**On the other hand ...**

*Table 8:* Setting my own experiment.

be anxious for the rest of the day because she'd had to do something that felt deeply unpleasant to her.

On the other hand, if the problem was one of her worrying about what might happen and how she would feel, as well as worrying about what other people might think or do, then it was likely that she'd feel anxious (because of her worry) – but also that nothing too bad would happen.

Chloe knew that if she thought she saw people looking at her, that didn't necessarily mean that they **were** staring. It also didn't mean that they were thinking unpleasant things about her. Again, it was a problem of her **worrying** about what people might think (**mind reading** was the thinking problem here).

Chloe found the experience quite difficult, but noted that nobody said anything unpleasant and that the barista in the coffee shop seemed friendly.

Chloe's **"one hand"** prediction didn't come true and she got some evidence that actually it might be a problem with her worrying about things, and not a problem with her appearance.

## ONE STEP AT A TIME

Whatever your experiment is, you can take smaller steps to make it easier, just like Chloe did. So if your experiment is to go on the bus, you might start with walking to the bus stop and waiting close by to see people getting on and off the bus, without getting on yourself. Then, on your first trip on the bus, you might just travel for one stop. But all the time you're doing these small steps, you're still challenging your thoughts, and taking in as much evidence about the experience as you can.

Now fill in this box with your own experience:

---

**Did the "one hand" prediction come true?**




**How did you feel?**




**If the "other hand" interpretation is that it is worry that is the problem, what does that mean for you now?**




**What do you conclude from this experiment?**



---

*Table 9: Analysing the outcome of the experiment.*

The likelihood is that, whatever you decide to do, it will not make you feel as anxious as you expect, but we don't know for certain. That is why it is an experiment!

So, over to you. How did you get on?

If you've answered honestly, you will probably have found that although the experience was scary, the 'one hand' prediction you've always told yourself would happen didn't actually happen. And we really hope that following on from that, you can see that actually, your **worry** about the thing happening is the driver for you and your anxiety, not your actual appearance.

Most of all, we hope that having done this once, you can do it again. But you will only be ready to do it again if you have been able to carry out your experiment in the right way. And that means letting go of safety behaviours ...

For example, let's say you're scared of crossing the road, so your friend suggests you do an experiment. The trouble is, you're so scared that you dash across the road extremely quickly, or you cross saying, 'Please don't die' to yourself over and over again.

This is a safety behaviour, just like keeping your eyes closed, avoiding the light in social situations, sitting furthest away from everyone on the bus etc. Behaviours like these will stop the experiment from being as effective as it could be.

So how can you tell if you're doing the experiment right?

Here's a good test for you: if the experiment feels too easy, it could mean that you're engaging in a safety behaviour! For example, let's say Chloe is doing an experiment in which she goes for a coffee at her local café without camouflaging her neck. If she doesn't wear her scarf, but wears a high-collared top and sits with her back against the wall, then she isn't doing the experiment right because she isn't truly exposing herself to the feared situation. She might say, 'Well, no one said anything because they couldn't really see my neck under my top, and I was hidden away from everyone else.' In other words, she wasn't really testing out whether someone might say something about her neck or not!

> **Remember – if you're trying an experiment, it will feel scary. It's supposed to feel a bit scary because that shows you that you're doing it right.**

Try to take each day as it comes. You will have bad days and blips. You will have days when it seems like you're not making any progress at all. But it's all part-and-parcel of any therapeutic process to have downs as well as ups. And the more you do your experiments, the more you'll be able to take on. It's like exercise. It feels hard at first when you haven't exercised for a long time. But the more you do it, the more you feel able to do it. And the more you achieve, the more you feel able to push yourself to achieve more.

## TESTING IT ALL OUT – SUMMARY

- To overcome your body image problem or BDD, you need to faceyour fear.

- To do this you need to set **experiments** for yourself, to test out what happens, and what interpretation (from the previous chapter) fits best.

- The more you do **experiments**, the easier they get.

- To do a fair experiment, you need to do it without any safety behaviours.

- **Habituation** helps you get used to the things that scare you. When you face a threat your anxiety spikes. But when you face a threat without safety behaviours you'll find that the anxiety reduces.

- When you try it, your experiment will feel scary. But that shows **you're doing it right** – without using old safety behaviours.

# SECTION 10

# MORE STRATEGIES TO HELP

## RUMINATION AND WORRY

Remember, rumination is the process of turning unhelpful thoughts over and over in your mind, either in the moment, or after the event. Worrying describes the process in which you devote excessive attention to potential future problems. Sometimes these terms can be used interchangeably and that's fine, as we can use the same strategies to help in both cases.

## WHY DO WE NEED TO STOP RUMINATING AND WORRYING?

Rumination and worry are not constructive processes. We cannot change things that have happened, nor can we predict things that will happen. So what's the point of them? They take up a lot of time, and they make us feel worse about ourselves and the things that have happened, as well as the things that haven't happened (and may never happen)!

Chloe struggled a lot with ruminating about past events, as well as worrying endlessly about future events. For example, at the time of writing, Chloe is preparing to be a bridesmaid at her sister's wedding. It's something she wants to do for her sister, but it's also something that she knows will be difficult. She will effectively be on display for several hours with no hiding place. That's quite a proposition for anybody with body image issues.

Chloe could quite easily devote hundreds of hours to worrying about it, but is that a constructive use of her time? If you devoted five hours, 10 hours, or even 200 hours to ruminating and worrying, are you going to be any closer to an answer? You can't possibly solve every possible permutation of events that could happen. You can't predict the outcome of any future event. If it hasn't happened, there isn't an answer waiting to be discovered.

One of the big issues with ruminating is that it can affect so much of your everyday life. There were many times when Chloe was talking to people when it was more important to her to evaluate how ugly she thought she looked, rather than concentrate on the conversation she was having. And then afterwards, she would ruminate about the conversation again and worry about how distracted she might have appeared.

You might also have noticed that, during a conversation, you're only able to devote some of your attention to what's being said, while most of your processing power focuses internally on:

- How you're feeling
- What you think you look like
- What the other person appears to be focusing on ...

It is like having two conversations at once – one in your own head, and the other with the person you're speaking to. How difficult is that?!

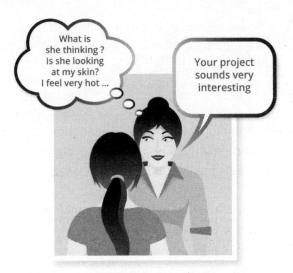

You might be able to nod and smile and be seemingly engaged in the conversation, but actually the more significant part of you would be evaluating what you've just said and how that relates to what the other person thinks of you. And then you get the double whammy – because you realise you've been stuck inside your own head and not really been listening, you become even more worried about the whole scenario. What did they say? Did you miss something important? Have they noticed that you aren't really focused? Do they think you're being rude? So, you see, ruminating in this scenario is not only unhelpful, it actually makes you worry more.

## HOW CAN RUMINATION AND WORRY AFFECT MOOD?

If you spend a lot of time at home going over things that have happened, again, you'll know that it can make you feel an awful lot worse. Let's try an experiment:

Spend 30 seconds thinking of something or somebody you love. It could be a favourite film or TV show, some music you love, playing a sport, or your favourite person. How did you feel after this?

Now spend 30 seconds thinking of something unpleasant, like a recent argument with a loved one, or when you last felt anxious about your appearance. How did you feel after this?

We strongly suspect you'll feel worse about the second example. But if we break it down, you know that the bad event has already happened, and nothing has changed. Even so, just thinking about things that have happened can affect your mood negatively, and can trap you in a vicious cycle of thoughts about something that can't even be changed.

*A-ha*, you might be thinking, *suppose thinking about bad things from the past stops them happening again in the future?* Others might think, *I really only want to worry about the important things. If I don't ruminate and worry about these things, I could be caught out. Or I could miss something that I hadn't considered.* There are two thinking problems at work here – **catastrophising** and **predicting the future**. You simply do not know what will happen in the future, and it's very, very unlikely that you will have an exact repeat of an event that has already happened! So this is not a fruitful way to spend your time. It will not change anything that has already happened and it will not change anything that might happen.

## It's time to stop!

So how do you stop ruminating or worrying? Well first, you need to know when you are doing it. Most people know when they get stuck in their heads, or they're spending too much time worrying. It is usually in trigger situations, after difficult events, or when thinking about things that might happen in the future. So, take a moment and list the times when you find yourself worrying or ruminating, or events that might trigger this process:

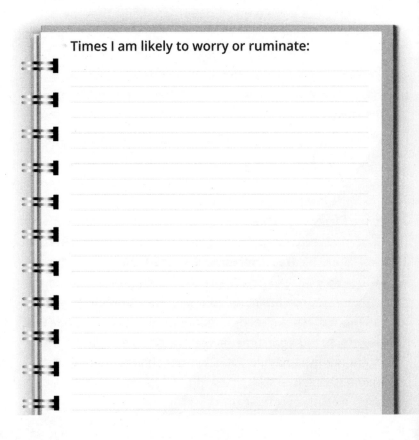

**Times I am likely to worry or ruminate:**

For example, Chloe was most likely to ruminate when she was in conversation with someone, or after speaking with people. She is most likely to worry about the prospect of being on show in some way in the future.

## ATTENTION RETRAINING

Now you have an idea of how and when ruminating and worrying are likely to be problems for you. As you know, ruminating and worrying both rely on you being in your head. You can't ruminate and worry and be fully engaged on an external task. It's just not possible. So, in order to stop ruminating and worrying you need to shift your attention from inside your head to outside your head – to what is going on around you.

Just so we're clear, this is different from avoidance / safety behaviour (which only reinforces the problem) because you are making a proactive decision to shift your attention on to something else; you're not doing it because you feel you have to. You can practise attention shifting anywhere so that, whenever you feel like you're fixating on your anxiety, or focusing on issues relating to your BDD, you can stop the unhelpful thoughts and re-focus your thinking.

## DEALING WITH WORRY

Inevitably, people with body image problems and BDD can get caught up in worrying about what might happen in the future, usually in a catastrophic way. They think about all the negative possibilities that could happen, and subsequently they find it hard to enjoy life. This kind of worry can prevent people from taking risks, just in case their worries become true.

This intense level of worry can really interfere in people's lives, so that they become totally caught up in unhelpful thinking patterns about the future and the many bad things they think might happen to them.

For example, when Chloe was working in the supermarket, she often worried that somebody would come over to her and ask her a question, and then she found it hard to concentrate on what she was doing because the thought of it scared her so much.

People sometimes think *I have to worry to stop bad things happening*. But worrying is an entirely unhelpful process if you are worrying about something you can't change. So you need to learn to spot the difference between worrying about something you can't solve and something you can solve. And here's how you can do that ...

Think of your problem and see which one of these scenarios it fits in:

**Scenario 1:** You don't know what is going to happen in the future and therefore you can't change what eventually happens.

**Scenario 2:** You know what's going to happen in the future and you still can't change what will happen.

**Scenario 3:** You know what will happen in the future and you can affect the outcome of it.

You will probably find that most, if not all of your worries will fit in Scenarios 1 and 2. We're sure you can accept that there is absolutely no point in worrying about things you cannot change, no matter how hard you try. Consequently, we can safely say that worrying about Scenarios 1 and 2 is a waste of your time.

So, if your worries fit in Scenario 1 and 2, we suggest discarding that line of thought, and if it helps, use some helpful distraction techniques.

## THE 'WHAT IF?' TREE

Another way of looking at worry is something we call the 'What if?' Tree. People who worry often ask themselves questions beginning with, 'What if …' and 'If only …' For example, Chloe used to think 'What if I could save up and have cosmetic surgery …'

You'll see that as soon as you start asking yourself, 'What if …?' or wondering 'If only …' your thoughts just circle round to more unanswerable questions. So how do you stop it?

You can **cut off the branch** of thought that starts with 'What if …' or 'If only …' by not answering the 'What if …' question. Here's an example:

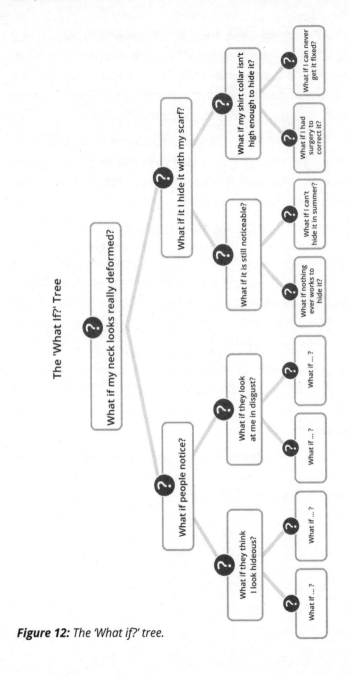

*Figure 12:* The 'What if?' tree.

You're having a very small get-together with your closest friends, when you hear a knock at the door. It's a friend of a friend – someone you really can't stand. Do you let them in and potentially ruin your evening?

The 'What if?' tree starts to tell you that it'd be unkind not to ask them in, you'll be considered rude, and you'll spend the evening feeling guilty. So you let the person in, and sure enough, you have a terrible time. You spend the whole evening thinking, 'If only I hadn't let them in.'

But, if you can cut out this branch – by telling the person that it wasn't a good time for you – you might feel anxious for a little while because it was an uncomfortable thing to do, but once you started enjoying the time with your friends, that feeling would reduce.

Of course, the earlier you cut the off the branch and stop trying to answer those impossible 'What if ...' questions, the sooner you'll forget them.

# OTHER HELPFUL STRATEGIES – SUMMARY

- Rumination is turning unhelpful thoughts over and over in your mind. Worrying applies to devoting excessive attention to future events. Ruminating and worrying do not make us feel any better. You cannot change the past, and you do not know what will happen in the future.

- Selective attention is when we scan our environment intently to pick up any potential threats and self-focused attention describes monitoring yourself to the exclusion of everything else

- To stop these unhelpful processes, you can **shift your attention** from inside your mind to what's going on around you.

- Stop trying to answer unanswerable 'What if ...' questions. **Cut off the branch** and let the feeling recede.

# SECTION 11

## APPEARANCE ISN'T EVERYTHING

One of the big issues we need to address with body image issues is the overvalued importance you put on your appearance to the exclusion of everything else.

Try to remember, you are more than just your appearance.

A healthy sense of self-worth isn't just based on appearance; it incorporates intelligence, sense of humour, abilities, interests, relationships and much more. But if you have body image problems, your sense of self-worth becomes heavily dependent on your appearance. This also means that your sense of self-worth will be very fragile and if you are unhappy with your appearance, your self-worth is badly affected. But if your sense of self-worth encompasses a broader range of attributes, it gives you a buffer for times when you have worries or feel uncomfortable about your appearance. It helps you to balance it against the other qualities that you value about yourself.

We have already suggested that you are more than just your appearance, but let's find a different way to think about this. We're going to use a pie chart to help you divide up what you value about yourself.

To give you an example, Chloe forgot so many of the things that made her who she was. Instead she was absolutely and utterly dominated by her perception of what she looked like. So, a pie chart depicting which components made up her sense of self would have looked like this:

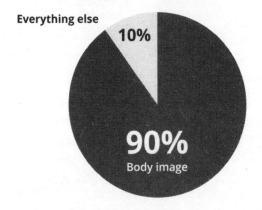

*Figure 13:* Chloe's pie chart before treatment.

As you can see, a huge 90% is dedicated to her appearance, leaving just 10% for all the other things that help define who she is: her sense of humour, her compassion, her friendships and family relationships, her hobbies and interests, her creativity, and her intellect. That really doesn't give a very accurate representation of Chloe as a person.

If we asked Chloe to give us another representation of her worth now though, this is what it might look like:

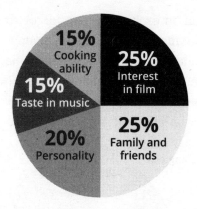

*Figure 14:* Chloe's pie chart after treatment.

Okay, now it's your turn. Show us how much you define yourself by your appearance at the moment, in the pie chart below. Don't worry if it's a lot! It doesn't make you vain or conceited, and we know you're working hard to put less emphasis on your appearance.

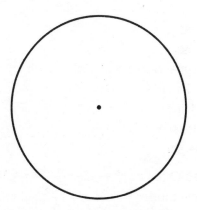

*Figure 15:* The value I give my appearance.

Now, take some time to think about all the other things about you that give you value as a person. It might be difficult to do, but focus on all those little things about you that make you interesting and unique and different. Think about the things that other people may have said they like about you – your sense of style, your dance moves, your knowledge of gardening etc.

Make a list of these things and give them a percentage value. Make sure you put "appearance" at the bottom of the list.

Do they all add up to 100%? If not, start at the top and work down again adjusting the values until they come out at 100%.

Now draw your new pie chart here:

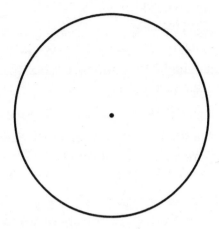

*Figure 16:* Things that make up my self-worth.

It can be hard to do this exercise and think about all the things that give us value as people, especially if you are used to being very self-critical. Another way to think about this is to think about what you would want people to say about you in a eulogy at your funeral. We know this sounds a bit morbid, but it can help focus your mind on how you would like to be remembered. Would you really like people to say you were overly concerned with how you looked and nothing else? Or would you prefer it if it incorporated all the things that make you a special person? We think it would be the latter.

There are a lot of wonderful and interesting things about you other than your appearance.

## SELF-CRITICISM

We've already mentioned self-criticism as a particularly unhelpful aspect of body image problems and BDD, and have labelled it a type of **thinking problem**. But actually, we are all self-critical from time to time. And initially that self-critical voice was intended to stop us embarrassing or humiliating ourselves in public. The problem is that, as we've seen, self-criticism can become pre-emptive and instead of staying silent for most of the time, it actually stays active in every situation.

For example, imagine you're going out after lunch. You'd want to check that you don't have any food stuck in your teeth, and your clothes are clean before you go. You don't want people to make any potentially embarrassing comments. So that little voice can actually be constructive when it comes to reminding us of the things we need to check in order to appear presentable.

But suppose this voice gets amplified and applied to every situation? The potentially helpful voice saying 'Do you look ready to go out?' turns into 'You don't look good enough. You'd better go and check in the mirror again.' So it becomes purely self-critical rather than helpful in any way. And if you're already dealing with worries associated with body image problems or BDD, it means you have to deal with a second wave of unhelpful thinking thanks to that self-critical voice.

So let's give you an exercise for seeing how destructive this self-critical voice can be.

Write down how you're feeling at the moment. Then, for 20 seconds, you are going to tell yourself that you are useless and terrible. Your criticisms could be related to your appearance, e.g. saying you're ugly, or they could be a form of criticism based on what you've been doing, e.g. 'Why did you say that?' or 'Why did you do that?'

Afterwards, write down how you're feeling. The likelihood is that you will obviously feel much worse about yourself, and a bit depressed.

Now, even if you don't believe the things you say, you are going to say positive things about yourself for 20 seconds. Afterwards, record how you feel.

Now, write down a list of positive, self-affirming statements, EVEN if you don't think they're true e.g. 'I'm a good person. I'm allowed to make mistakes just like everybody else. I'm not perfect, but I am good enough. I'm good at basketball, I am a good friend,' etc. If you think you'll have trouble coming up with self-affirming statements off-the-cuff, ask a relative or a friend – we're sure they'll be very happy to help you.

So how did it go?

It's very likely that you're going to feel much more positive after the second exercise. This proves what an impact your being self-critical can have – having that negative parrot on your shoulder makes you feel worse about yourself, and that makes it much easier to get caught up in unhelpful thinking patterns around BDD and body image problems.

But it also means that positive statements can be empowering. So what we would like you to do is keep them to hand. Print them off and put them in your bag, purse, or wallet, keep them on your phone, or record them as an audio file on your phone. Then you can listen to them whenever you find that self-critical voice popping up, or even just a couple of times a day, regardless of how you feel. In fact, we would recommend reading or listening to these positive statements at least twice a day. And you can continue to add positive statements to the list as you think of them, or whenever other people say nice things to you.

## GETTING OBJECTIVE INFORMATION WITH SURVEYS

It can also help to use surveys to help you challenge unhelpful beliefs. For example, it might be that someone, a man, is convinced that their black hair / height / jaw shape is hideously unattractive. Consequently, they also believe that this one aspect of their appearance is the most important feature that potential partners would consider. In this situation, we would design and carry out a survey to find out what people actually think. For example:

1. What aspects / characteristics do you consider attractive in men? Please list them below in the order you find them most attractive.

2. What hair colour do you look for in partners?

3. What height would you want your perfect partner to be?

4. What characteristics or qualities do you look for in a partner?

A survey generates a whole range of responses, and that can provide a useful insight into how other people actually think.

Have a think about what you would ask if you were to undertake a survey? What beliefs would you like to test out? What questions would I ask?

Then think about who you would ask? You can always get a friend or family member to do the survey for you if you feel too embarrassed. We would recommend getting at least 10 responses – but the more responses the better! Then you have a lot more data to think about.

## SELECTIVE ATTENTION AND SELF-FOCUSED ATTENTION

People with body image issues usually have problems with **selective attention**. This means that they scan their environment for potential threats (in other words, they selectively attend to information in their environment that has the potential to be threatening). An example of this would be scanning the room for reflective surfaces or mirrors to ensure you can check your appearance, or scanning other people's faces to see if they have noticed that something is wrong with your appearance. Perhaps you've noticed yourself doing these things. If you have, then you know that living life in a hyper-vigilant state, constantly scanning for threats, is tiring and takes your attention away from enjoying the moment.

**Self-focused attention** is when you spend time monitoring yourself, your feelings, and your responses, to the exclusion of other things. You may remember that Chloe would do this when she was talking to someone, and then realised that she was so busy monitoring herself and how she felt that she lost focus on the conversation. Further, she worried about whether she had missed something that was said, or if the other person had noticed her being a bit absent from the conversation.

Another problem with self-focused attention is that if you're monitoring yourself constantly, you will find something to worry about! Think about it, if you spend 30 seconds just appraising how you're feeling, noticing everything about yourself and your body, you will find something to worry about. It could be a spot on your face, or a pain in your leg, or how you're feeling. You wouldn't have noticed it before, but now that you have, it is hard to un-notice it – and then it can often feed into your anxiety.

Now, we've said that the more attention you give to something, whether it is self-focused, or scanning the environment for threats, the more it will hold us in its grip. So, one way of stopping this from happening is to shift your attention to something external and something less threatening.

Here's an exercise to demonstrate how that works.

> Take exactly one minute to focus in on the aspect of your appearance or the event that most worries you. Set a timer on your phone so you know when a minute is up.
>
> As soon as the minute is up, look at the picture below and spend between 30 seconds and one minute describing it in as much detail as you possibly can. Say the things out loud.

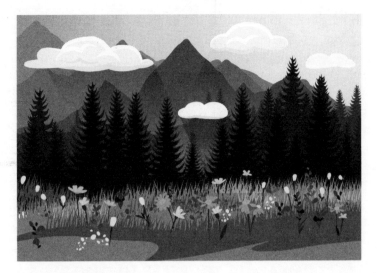

How did you get on?

We predict that you probably felt extremely anxious after a minute focusing in on your body image issues, but shifting your attention to something else will hopefully have distracted you. As a result, your anxiety will have lessened considerably.

When we do this in therapy with people, pretty much everyone says they quickly forgot about the aspect of their appearance or the event that was worrying them. The interesting thing about this is that the level of threat (i.e. your appearance or what other people might be thinking) has not actually changed at all. What has changed is the level of attention you've been paying to it – and that strongly suggests that ...

> **The amount of attention you pay to your perceived problem only makes your anxiety worse**

Now have another go at the exercise. But this time, try to do the second part of the exercise in your head, so that next time, it will be easier for you to do it in public. Saying the things in your head does feel a bit harder at first, but it will get easier with practice, to the point you will be able to do it any time and any place. You won't have the picture with you when you're out and about, but you can find something else. For example, you could focus in on people's shoes and note all the colours, or spot how many red things you can see in the street, or keep track of how many shops you've passed with the letter G in the shop name.

## COMPARING YOURSELF TO OTHERS

If you find yourself going online and comparing yourself to the images of people on Facebook and Instagram and comparing your features, it can feel difficult to stop! You're probably aware that this is a very unhelpful thing to do – and it isn't a fair basis for comparison. You'll only be looking at images of people who are posting really happy and smiley images of themselves on holiday, or having fun. Very often these pictures will have been touched up afterwards, or taken with a special app or a filter. You need to remember that people posting their photos online will have hand-picked the images as being really good representations of them at their best. It is much less common for people to post the unflattering images in the wrong light, or when they're not feeling their best. They will have selectively edited out images of their double chin, or chosen the best angle of their nose. In other words, these images are not realistic representations of a person, or their life.

Anyway, would you really want the whole of your person and your life judged by one photo? We certainly wouldn't, as it wouldn't convey the richness and complexity of ourselves and our lives.

We suggest that you take a break from the social media sites you use to compare yourself – or at least limit yourself to ten minutes a day. Most of all, please don't use them at all if you're feeling particularly vulnerable or sad. There is nothing helpful to be gleaned from viewing these images, and in fact, you might find something infinitely more useful to do with your time instead.

Similarly, if you compare yourself with people you see on the street, you're probably only comparing yourself in a very selective way – picking out the people you consider to be very attractive, or the ones who have a particular feature that you think is ideal (if you're comparing specific bodily features) and just ignoring the rest. This very biased 'screening' process only helps to confirm your unhelpful beliefs about yourself.

If you're comparing yourself in public, and you know that you're being biased about who you're looking at, try to widen your focus, so that you look at absolutely everybody to give you a more representative data set.

Alternatively, shift your focus and change your attention. Because this comparing process is very unhelpful, it will most likely make you feel more anxious and sad. So as soon as you realise you're scanning everybody's nose, or their forehead, or whatever it is that you're fixating on, shift your attention to their shoes.

## AVOIDANCE OR DISTRACTION?

We've talked a bit in this chapter about avoidance and distraction and it's worth clarifying the difference. If you say, 'I am not going to deal with this; I'll just ignore it,' that's avoidance. But distraction is owning the problem and dealing with it by choosing to do something else: 'I understand and ACCEPT that this is making me feel this way, and I am just ruminating / worrying about it; so instead I am choosing to think about something else.' By making an active choice, you are still acknowledging the difficult feelings and thinking processes, but you choose to do something else while the feelings subside and to help you stop thinking unhelpfully. If you are using distraction, you may still feel anxious or have the occasional unhelpful thought about your appearance creep in, and that's okay because distraction is not meant to suddenly make things perfect. But it allows you to step away from the intensity of the anxiety and unhelpful thinking, until they reduce to a more comfortable level.

You can choose whichever distractions you think will help you most. It could be a simple repetitive task like tidying or exercise. You might enjoy cooking or reading, or perhaps you find it easier to divert unhelpful thoughts when you watch a film. Choose whatever works for you.

## COPING WITH UNCOMFORTABLE
## AND DISTRESSING FEELINGS

Strong emotional states like anxiety, frustration, low mood, and sadness are inevitable parts of life and we all experience them, to varying degrees, from time to time. But if you have been dealing with body image issues and BDD, then you know the emotions you experience can be extremely distressing and disabling. One of the main reasons why body image issues are so hard to deal with though is because our safety behaviours are designed to avoid these difficult feelings. That's normal, right? After all, if you were experiencing physical pain, you'd try to identify the source of the pain and then move away from it. If the hot water tap burns your hand, you take your hand away.

But emotional pain is quite different. Avoidance from emotional pain is not the answer. If you avoid it, it will find a way to creep back in some way. And as soon as your avoidance strategy has ended, the emotional pain will be there waiting once again. Accepting, managing, and tolerating your strong emotions – even the terrifying ones – is the key.

Unfortunately, society is geared up to the quick-fix. We're taught to believe that feeling uncomfortable is wrong and that if we have even the slightest twinge of an unpleasant emotion, we need to "solve" it immediately. For example, if your train is delayed by a few minutes, you feel the frustration for the delay. You expect things to happen straightaway. We're misinformed that life should be perfect, but it isn't. It can't be. And there's nothing we can do to fix a lot of the sad and difficult things that happen – other than try to process what we feel about these things, learn from the experience, and then move on.

## FACING OUR EMOTIONS

Our maddening, conflicting and frequently confusing emotions all help mark us out as being truly human. When someone we love dies, we grieve for them. But we don't grieve with the same intensity forever. Over time our grief fades, and while we know things might never be the same again without that person in our life, life assumes a new "normal".

Even when our emotions are distressing and intense, we know that they won't always stay that way. They will have to change sometime. Whenever you have felt incredibly anxious, that feeling of anxiety did reduce. Maybe not immediately, but eventually it did. This is what we call the Law of Impermanence. No emotional state is permanent.

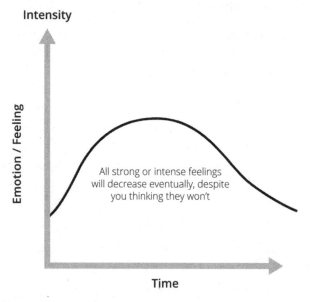

*Figure 17: Impermanence of emotions.*

You will see that your anxiety level will rise in a tough situation, but the level of intensity will eventually drop. All emotions, regardless of how intense they are or how frequently they occur, will reduce.

Just think about how you were feeling when you got up this morning, or when you first picked up this book, or even when you had lunch. Your feelings now will be different. Even if you were feeling low and you still feel low, the intensity of that feeling will probably have changed.

Just knowing this can be a real game changer for a lot of people who think that they are mired in the same emotional state every hour of every day of their lives. Clearly, the degrees of difference may be very much smaller if you are experiencing severe depression, but there will still be differences nonetheless.

This means (and we know this can be hard to believe when you are living with severe anxiety or depression) that neither your pleasant or unpleasant feelings will last for ever.

## APPEARANCE ISN'T EVERYTHING – SUMMARY

- Your self-worth isn't defined by your appearance. It's made up of all those things that make you special and **unique**.

- Surveys are a good way to collect data to check out what other people think about appearance.

- **Positive self statements** can help to remind us of all the positive things about ourselves and help to overcome self-criticism.

# SECTION 12

# CALM BODY, CALM MIND

When you start to use the strategies we've talked about more and more, you'll have the reassurance of knowing that there are measures you can take when body image symptoms strike. But what happens if they don't work? Everyone who has ever been in recovery from body image issues will have had times when nothing seems to work. *Hang on,* you think, *I'm doing everything my therapist told me, or I'm following the strategies in the book, but it's just not working!* So why is that?

Remember earlier, we talked about the times when your body goes into fight, flight or freeze mode? When that happens it changes your body chemistry – the stress hormones adrenaline, norepinephrine and cortisol flood your body – and it takes a full half hour for the effects to die down. It's like suddenly being flooded with alcohol; you can't just switch off the effects. And so of course, it is much, much harder to stay calm and logical when your body is on high alert, ready to tackle a perceived threat. Although it may feel like your strategies to challenge your thinking aren't working, that isn't the case. It's just that while your body is in threat mode, it's harder for your mind to listen to what you're saying. That part of your brain will not work in the same way if you're in threat mode; cognitive challenging won't work in that moment.

So what do you do to get through moments of extreme body image-related stress? Let's say you wake up and already feel sick to your stomach with stress and anxiety; that means you won't be in any state to try a behavioural exercise.

Here are some suggestions for you – try them all and assess them to see which ones work to reduce your baseline stress levels. It's important that you try them when you don't have any anxiety so that you already know what to do when your anxiety starts to rise. If you wait until you're already experiencing anxiety to see if they work, it'll be too late.

### Effective breathing

Let's start with your breathing. Don't underestimate just how valuable effective breathing can be. Here is a breathing exercise to help you.

Count to four as you breathe in, then count to six as you breathe out. Close your eyes, clear your mind, and focus on your breathing. One of the first things that usually happens when you start to panic is that your breathing speeds up, so concentrating on exhaling for six seconds can help calm you down. The outward breath releases tension in the chest too. Don't forget to try this at home when you're already feeling quite calm and then practise it more and more so you can use it in increasingly stressful situations.

## Exercise

Getting a little bit of exercise is good for the mind and body, and releases lots of endorphins which will help you feel better. If you can get some fresh air at the same time, even better. You don't have to do anything strenuous to get the benefits of exercise – a walk in the park is absolutely fine.

Sometimes the activity and the change of scenery is enough to occupy your mind in a more positive way, but if it isn't, try challenging yourself to spot things beginning with every letter of the alphabet, or see how many red things you can spot ... these are all good ways to distract your attention and help your stress levels return to normal.

## Mindfulness

This is a great way to shift attention from your internal world to the external world. Engage your senses; see the clouds, feel the grass, breathe in the rich aromas of the coffee shop – do whatever you can to engage your senses and focus on living in the here-and-now.

Mindfulness teaches you to experience every situation as it is, rather than how you think it is, or how you want it to be. And then, when your mind wanders so that you notice other thoughts creeping back in, you bring your attention back to the moment in hand.

One of the reasons why mindfulness is such a good technique to practise is that it takes judgement out of the equation. When you're being mindful, you learn to accept whatever thoughts and feelings you have without questioning them or trying to analyse them.

### Helpful distraction

Distraction techniques can be very useful too. But please bear in mind that doing something to distract you isn't going to give you complete relief, nor is it intended to. You are learning to acknowledge the anxiety, knowing that it will reduce in intensity. See more on helpful distraction in Section 5.

## What works best for you?

See which techniques make a positive difference, keep referring to them, and incorporate them into your daily routine.

When your body feels a bit calmer, you can then get started with your thought challenging techniques. They'll feel much more effective now.

# CALM BODY, CALM MIND – SUMMARY

- When the body goes into fight, flight or freeze mode, stress hormones flood your body – which makes it difficult to process information rationally.

- To reduce your baseline stress, you can practise effective breathing, exercise, mindfulness techniques and distraction exercises.

- It is a good idea to practise these techniques in non-threatening situations first, then you can use them in anxiety provoking situations.

- When your body feels calmer, you can move on to thought challenging exercises.

# SECTION 13

## MENTAL IMAGERY

Using mental imagery techniques can be very helpful, particularly for those with a diagnosis of BDD, but anyone with body image problems can benefit from using these strategies.

We're going to tell you about a mental imagery re-scripting technique to help you look at any difficult experiences relating to your appearance or body image that have happened in the past. These experiences may have been embarrassing, humiliating, shaming or traumatic and they may have all contributed to the built-up felt impressions and beliefs that you have about yourself, your appearance and your body.

Let's start by looking at an example scenario:

At age 13, having just started secondary school, some boys teased Evie and said she had a big nose. That was a traumatic experience for Evie, particularly at such a young and impressionable age, and it got stuck in her head. In other words, she wasn't able to deal with the unpleasant feelings and move on without letting it affect her any more. Whether or not she had a big nose by an objective measure is irrelevant. The shame and embarrassment she felt meant that the experience really stuck with her, and as a result, a preoccupation with her nose started to build up from this point.

Even though Evie is now in her thirties, the experience of 13-year-old Evie has really stuck with her. Because she was unable to process them properly at the time, those feelings still flash up, and she continues to be very concerned about the size of her nose.

Mental imagery is a way of building a bridge between then and now. It can help you to update the old experiences, based on what you know now. For example, Evie now understands that it isn't her nose that's the problem, it's the way she worries about it. While it was obviously a devastating experience, Evie also now knows that her nose is not the most important feature about her. She recognises that it's okay to have features that she doesn't like and it doesn't mean that the feature she dislikes makes her hideous and ugly. However, she still feels that her nose is too big (**emotional reasoning**) and feels very anxious in a number of different scenarios because she worries about the size of her nose.

So now, grown up Evie needs a way to let the 13-year old Evie know what she knows. If she can do that, it can help her deal with the difficult emotions and worries about her nose. So mental imagery can help you update these old experiences, and hopefully reduce their interference in your life today.

Mental imagery techniques are not meant to undo any bad experiences. They're meant to update them with the more helpful information that you didn't have at the time, or you weren't aware of. So it isn't about pretending that an experience didn't happen. It did happen. But what we've taken from the experience, emotionally and cognitively, isn't very helpful, and doesn't really fit the facts.

If you'd had more information at that time, or you'd had someone who could point out a better way to think about it, you would have been able to deal with it in a healthier way.

## USING MENTAL IMAGERY

To start with, you need to identify any relevant past experiences that relate to your body image and appearance. There might be just one, or a few. If you can't think of a historical event, you can use a more recent example of a time where you felt embarrassed or mortified about your appearance.

When you've identified this experience, describe it here using the **present tense** – as if it is happening to you right now. It is important to include any thoughts that you had, how you felt emotionally, how you felt in your body, and what you did (if anything). Here's an example:

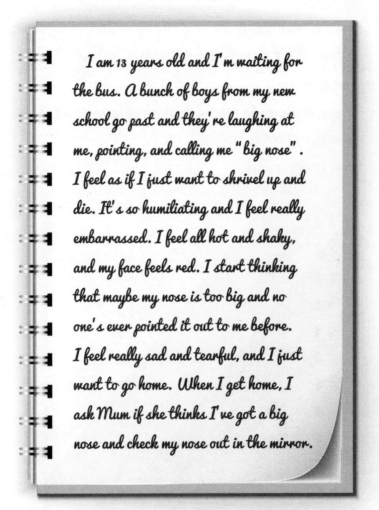

*I am 13 years old and I'm waiting for the bus. A bunch of boys from my new school go past and they're laughing at me, pointing, and calling me "big nose". I feel as if I just want to shrivel up and die. It's so humiliating and I feel really embarrassed. I feel all hot and shaky, and my face feels red. I start thinking that maybe my nose is too big and no one's ever pointed it out to me before. I feel really sad and tearful, and I just want to go home. When I get home, I ask Mum if she thinks I've got a big nose and check my nose out in the mirror.*

You'll see how Evie has written this as it is happening to her now. She has also included:

Her thoughts and feelings: *"I think I have a big nose."*

Her emotions:

*"It's so humiliating and I feel really embarrassed."*

How she felt in her body:

*"I feel all hot and shaky and my face feels red."*

What she did:

*"I ask Mum if she thinks I've got a big nose and check my nose out in the mirror."*

**Now, it's your turn:**

Well done! It can be hard to think about these experiences and write them down. Please note, if it brings up any really distressing feelings for you – and you find them hard to deal with – take some time and use some of the strategies in the coping with distressing feelings chapter. You can come back to this when you feel more settled.

After writing about your experience, identify the unhelpful thoughts and beliefs from that experience, e.g. Evie's belief that she had a big nose. It may be about a specific feature like Evie's example, or your appearance in general, 'I'm ugly, or it could be more general, e.g. 'I'm unlovable'. Note these beliefs down here:

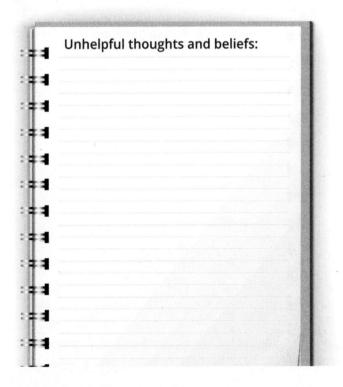

**Unhelpful thoughts and beliefs:**

Now we need to challenge these beliefs using the thought challenging techniques that you've learned in this book from chapter, e.g. identifying and changing unhelpful thinking patterns, and the Two Hands Thinking Technique.

Evie took her belief – *I have a big nose* – and, using the Two Hands Thinking Technique, came up with the more helpful and realistic belief that *I am worried that I had a big nose because I was teased when I was younger. But actually, the problem is my worrying about it.*

What are your more helpful interpretations?

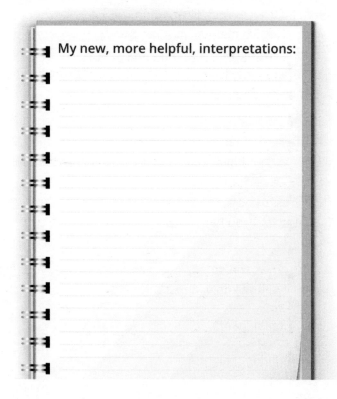

**My new, more helpful, interpretations:**

## TAKE YOURSELF BACK

It would have been helpful to have these updated, more constructive beliefs when you were younger. It would have been much easier for the younger version of you to stop the experience from interfering in the development of unhelpful beliefs about yourself and your appearance.

It was helpful to have the grown-up Evie visit younger Evie in her memory, and tell her that things were going to be okay. She would tell young Evie that it wasn't just her that the boys were picking on that day – they were pointing at everyone from school and saying random things about their appearance. They didn't know the full impact of their actions. She also needed younger Evie to know that there is nothing wrong with her nose, and she'll grow up to be a very interesting, lovely person with good friends, good relationships, and lots of potential.

Have a think about what else the younger version of you really needs in that moment. Would it be helpful for the younger you to have someone to tell you that things will be okay? Or perhaps you'd just want someone to give you a hug? Would you want your mum to be there? Or maybe it would it help if you had an older version of you to explain things?

Write down the things you would want the younger version of you to know in that moment:

## So how do you take yourself back?

First, close your eyes and take some deep breaths. When you feel relaxed, revisit the experience. For example, you're back at the bus stop, or wherever you were when the incident happened.

Going back in your memory like this is a bit like being the director of the movie of your life.

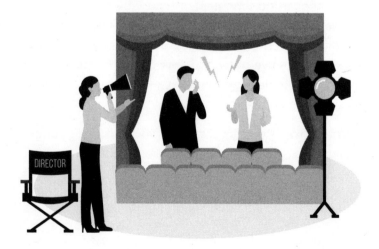

You run through the experience as it happened in reality, and then edit it. What does the younger version of you need? Perhaps she needs some soothing and some support. You can pause the video at the key moment and zoom in. So when the boys are mean and laugh at you, you can bring in the older version of you, or your mum, or someone else who will take your hand, give you a hug and tell you those helpful things. They'll reassure you that your nose isn't bigger or smaller than normal, and that the boys are teasing everyone else too. Then carry on the experience in your head so that you get on the bus with your mum, the older version of you, or whoever you've brought along to help you.

> **At the end of the experience, you need to finish up feeling secure, comfortable, and most importantly, safe.**

You might find it helpful to write down the updated experience here. You can also read it out loud and record it, and then listen back to it so you can re-experience the new, more positive outcome every time you listen. It will also be a good idea to repeat this exercise for any of the emotionally painful experiences in your past.

Give it a try to see how you get on.

**My experience:**

Well done for giving this a go! This exercise can be quite demanding, so if you feel tired or a bit out of sorts afterwards, please do something nice and compassionate for yourself afterwards. For example, watch a favourite film or take a gentle walk. It will let the experience settle down emotionally. And it's good to give yourself a break and enjoy some quality time after being brave enough to give this a go.

## MENTAL IMAGERY – SUMMARY

- Mental imagery is a way of building a bridge between the past and the present.

- It is a way of updating past experiences with the new information you didn't have before.

- Mental imagery or re-scripting is particularly important for people who have clear memories of events that relate to their unhelpful beliefs about themselves and their appearance, for example being teased for the way you look.

- It is not the same as saying the event didn't happen, happen. You're simply using all the knowledge and understanding you have now (which you didn't have then) to make it easier to process.

# SECTION 14

# DEPRESSION AND MEDICATION

It's perfectly normal to experience clinical depression as a result of body image problems and BDD. You will remember that Chloe experienced co-morbid depression – that is depression that occurs alongside BDD or body image problems.

It's important to clarify that here we are discussing depression as a result of body image problems and BDD. Depression that already existed before these issues may require separate treatment, which is not covered in this book. If that is the case for you, we recommend that you see your doctor for further advice. You will also find more help on dealing with depression at www.shawmindfoundation.org.

**We define Major Depressive Disorder as a low mood that lasts for more than two weeks, plus five of the following symptoms:**

- Feeling tearful and hopeless
- Reduced interest in pleasurable activities
- Significant weight gain or loss
- Insomnia or hypersomnia (sleeping too little or too much)

- Sluggishness

- Feeling tired

- Loss of energy

- Feeling worthless or excessively guilty

- Not being able to think

- Inability to concentrate or make decisions

- Thoughts of suicide[17]

We may all experience some of these symptoms from time to time, so if you think you've been experiencing five or more symptoms for two weeks or more, we do recommend you see your doctor.

Understandably, some people find thoughts of suicide worrying and frightening. Perhaps you think, or have previously thought, that you don't deserve to be around any more. Or perhaps you've wondered if people would be better off without you in their lives. You might have even felt that you simply can't cope with life any more. While it is not uncommon to have suicidal thoughts, as clinicians, we would be concerned if you are finding comfort in the thought of killing yourself, if you have made a plan to kill yourself, or if you have tried to kill yourself in the past. In any of these cases, we would ask you to seek direct professional help straightaway from your doctor or the emergency services. You may also be able to talk to your family or friends. For further information please visit: www.theshawmindfoundation.org

People who live with body image problems and BDD can suffer with other depression issues, including Persistent Depressive Disorder (which used to be called Dysthymic Disorder). This is a persistent, but slightly less severe, low mood that lasts for most of the day, and occurs more frequently than it doesn't, for at least two years. Sufferers do not have a reprieve from these symptoms for longer than two months in those two years. The symptoms of Dysthymic Disorder may not be as severe as Major Depressive Disorder, but the disorder is chronic and constant. Alongside the low mood, you will experience two of the following symptoms: low appetite, low energy, low self-esteem, poor concentration, feelings of hopelessness, and difficulty making decisions.[18]

Both these depressive disorders are debilitating in their own right, but they can also affect the process of recovery from body image problems and BDD. You can appreciate that if you're feeling depressed, it will affect your appetite and your ability to sleep, and that is going to dampen your motivation. In other words, depression will make it much, much harder to overcome your body image issues. But the good news is that working through the treatment strategies outlined in this programme can help lift your depression over time.

## MEDICATION FOR DEPRESSION

In terms of the treatment process, we would consider whether the person might benefit from medication. A lot of the medication used to treat obsessional and anxiety-related illness is also prescribed for depression, and if you're co-morbidly depressed, it might be helpful for you to speak with a medical specialist about what medication might be appropriate for you. This could provide the boost and the extra impetus you need to help you to start getting better.

Research suggests medication can be a useful way to kick-start recovery in most cases. If someone had a physical illness or an ongoing medical condition like diabetes, no one would question the value of medication. However, medication solely on its own will not always lead to recovery from depression – so we would still encourage you to follow the methods outlined in this programme to complement the benefits from medication.

## OTHER STRATEGIES

What else can you do to combat the effects of depression?

One of the first things that happens when people get depressed is that they stop doing many or all of the things they used to enjoy. Perhaps you used to meet up with your friends every week, or take part in a team sport, or maybe you used to go out with your colleagues after work – depression puts a stop to all of that. It takes away your motivation and to some extent your enjoyment, so typically, you simply retreat to your home to be alone. It gets to the point where just the thought of getting up and doing something can seem utterly exhausting. As the depression depletes your energy and takes the pleasure out of the things you used to do, it starts its own vicious cycle of inactivity: you don't put any effort into things, and consequently, you get nothing back. So to remedy this, we need to give you **behaviour booster**.[19]

Let's take a look at one of the activities you used to enjoy before depression set in, using a scale to chart the relationship between the effort you put in and the enjoyment you got out. We'll use the example of going swimming.

## BEFORE DEPRESSION

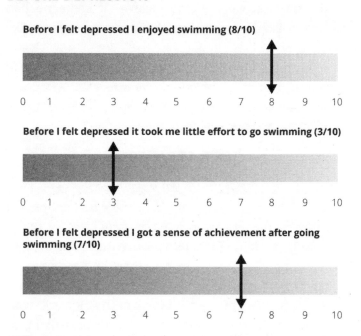

**Before I felt depressed I enjoyed swimming (8/10)**

0   1   2   3   4   5   6   7   8   9   10

**Before I felt depressed it took me little effort to go swimming (3/10)**

0   1   2   3   4   5   6   7   8   9   10

**Before I felt depressed I got a sense of achievement after going swimming (7/10)**

0   1   2   3   4   5   6   7   8   9   10

*Figure 18:* Enjoyment, effort and sense of achievement before depression.

You'll see that you scored 8/10 on the Scale One (the "Enjoyment" scale), and it just took a little effort (3/10) to motivate yourself to go swimming.

Now, let's see what happens to the numbers if we evaluate the enjoyment you got from swimming you were in the middle of an episode of depression.

## DURING A DEPRESSED EPISODE

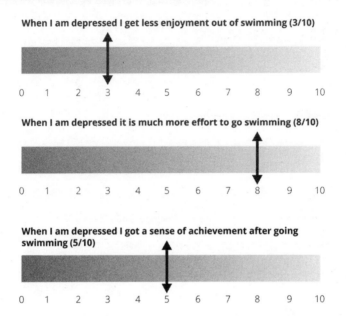

**When I am depressed I get less enjoyment out of swimming (3/10)**

0    1    2    3    4    5    6    7    8    9    10

**When I am depressed it is much more effort to go swimming (8/10)**

0    1    2    3    4    5    6    7    8    9    10

**When I am depressed I got a sense of achievement after going swimming (5/10)**

0    1    2    3    4    5    6    7    8    9    10

**Figure 19:** *Enjoyment, effort and sense of achievement before depression.*

By this stage, the depression has you in such a strong grip that the scale has effectively been reversed. You get very little enjoyment from meeting your friend, or from any other activity, and the effort it takes to get out is now much greater.

So there's little wonder that people stop doing the things they enjoy when it takes so much effort for such a small reward.

So if we examine the situation now, in the middle of depression, let's see what happens when you simply avoid going swimming:

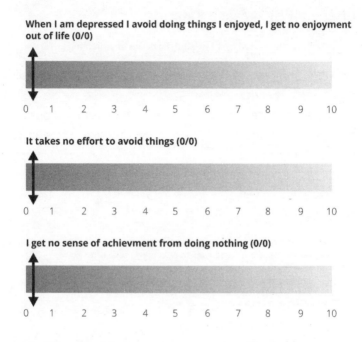

**When I am depressed I avoid doing things I enjoyed, I get no enjoyment out of life (0/0)**

0  1  2  3  4  5  6  7  8  9  10

**It takes no effort to avoid things (0/0)**

0  1  2  3  4  5  6  7  8  9  10

**I get no sense of achievment from doing nothing (0/0)**

0  1  2  3  4  5  6  7  8  9  10

***Figure 20:*** *Effect of avoidance on enjoyment, effort and sense of achievement.*

The depression has you in such a strong grip that you are not getting any enjoyment or much of a sense of achievement from swimming or any other activity, so you avoid it, as you are not getting any enjoyment or feeling effective at all! But look again at Figure 19. Are you able to extract that little bit of enjoyment, despite the effort you have to make, to go swimming? If you at least make the effort, you are highly likely to find that it wasn't as bad as you thought, and that you maybe even got more than 3/10 along the enjoyment scale. This is much better than 0/10 on the scale. Similarly, you will still get a sense of achievement from going swimming, even if you swim half the distance you used to.

We have found that this **behaviour booster** is an excellent way to refocus people's beliefs about the relationship between effort and enjoyment. While you might experience less enjoyment from your favourite activities than you're used to, **any enjoyment is still better than none**. As we have seen with other techniques in this book, the more you do it, the easier it gets, and the more effective it will be. So using this scale can be a useful motivational tool.

From this, we can devise a diary in which you plan a few activities ahead. Don't plan anything too heavy or too taxing, but instead focus on little things that will help you reconnect with the things you used to enjoy, or give you more of an empowered, useful feeling. Be prepared for the obstacles that lie ahead. Note them down now so you can work out a way of dealing with them in advance.

In the box below, fill in some activities that you used to enjoy, or gave you a sense of usefulness.

## My activities this week are ...

**Table 10:** *Design your own behaviour booster.*

I plan to do these activities on the following days at the following time (e.g. Wednesday afternoon)

After the activity describe how it went below. How much effort did it take? How much enjoyment did you get from it? Did you get a sense of achievement?

**What obstacles did you overcome in order to complete this activity?**

**Mark your rating from 1 to 10**

Enjoyment ___   Effort ___   Achievement ___

Another way of examining depression is to look at **thinking problems**. You'll remember that earlier, we looked at the ways thinking problems such as **catastrophising** and **mind reading** can relate to body image problems, and they can also apply to depression. For example, saying 'Oh, I can't be bothered to meet my friend tonight. It's going to take me ages to get ready and they'll think I'm boring because I've not been out of the house since I saw them last week.' Inevitably, if you think like that, you'll find it very hard to muster the enthusiasm to go.

**A better way of examining this way of thinking is to question it:**

- Is it 100% true that there is no point in going out tonight?
  *No. You haven't done it yet, so you can't possibly know what the outcome will be.*

- Is it helpful to think about it this way?
  *No, because it's stopping me from doing things.*

Any element of doubt opens up the possibility of looking at the situation in another way. So instead, you could perhaps say to yourself, 'Okay, I do still have some bad days, but friends tell me I'm making progress. They've been really supportive, and I do feel better after I've seen them.'

Again, we can use the **Two Hands Thinking Technique** to interpret a situation. You can choose to go with your first explanation, or you can choose to see it a different way that might actually be a truer representation of the situation.

**In any difficult situation, ask yourself:**

- Is my interpretation 100% accurate?
- Is this a helpful way to think?
- Am I giving in to any thinking problems?
- Is there another way I can interpret the situation, e.g. 'On the one hand … / on the other hand … ?'

Just remember, you don't have to make the new way of thinking about the situation sound perfect. Life isn't perfect. Things are frequently more difficult than we would like. But you can reflect this in your new way of thinking, e.g. *I know I am feeling low, and that makes it feel like hard work going out.*

*But there is a chance I'll enjoy it – even if just a little bit – and that probably means it's worth the effort to go.*

## MEDICATION

It's worth talking about medication (specifically for treating BDD) briefly at this point. Of course, there is no one-size-fits-all solution, and not everyone will benefit from medication. Indeed, current advice does not automatically recommend medication for the treatment of body image issues or BDD. And in some cases, a good course of psychological treatment based on CBT can be an effective treatment on its own.

However, some people with moderate to severe BDD, or with co-morbid depression, might require medication to help lift their mood or help their treatment to progress, particularly in the early stages. This also applies in cases where people don't meet the diagnostic criteria for BDD, but whose body image issues still cause low mood and depression. If you have BDD or a more severe body image problem which causes depression, evidence shows that medication is likely to help you alongside a good course of psychological treatment.[20]

The Selective Serotonin Re-uptake Inhibitors (SSRI) family of medication has been proven to be effective for anxiety, BDD and depression, and is often the first choice for people suffering with anxiety or obsessive related illness.

The type of medication prescribed will depend on individual factors including medication history and medical background, and the prescribed doses will vary within a recommended range. Sometimes doctors may even combine medications if it is clinically indicated. Antidepressant medications are not addictive, and there is good evidence that they can help in cases of BDD, anxiety, and depression.

> We suggest you talk to your doctor about the available options and the possible side effects of different kinds of medication.

Just because side effects are possible, it doesn't mean that you will necessarily get any of them; everyone responds to medication differently. And if one particular drug doesn't work for you, another one might, so don't worry if you don't respond positively to the first medication you try. The effects of many possible side effects tend to fade within the first three weeks.

There are some misconceptions about the role medication can play in treatment.

Some people might think that they only got better solely because of the medication, but that isn't usually the case. The complexity of body image problems or BDD means that the hard work you undertake in following a course of evidence-based treatment, like this one, is absolutely essential.

There will also be people who believe they are "weak" if they are prescribed medication, believing it means that they cannot get over their psychological problems on their own. Again, not true. We wouldn't tell anyone to stop taking medication for a physical illness, and the same holds true if you have been prescribed medicine for BDD, body image issues or depression. While we don't definitively understand the roots of body image problems, there may be biological factors at play, making medication a necessary part of a treatment plan. In Chloe's case, a blend of the right medication and the compassionate approach to understanding, embracing and dealing with her feelings was very effective.

So, in short, review the options for medication with your doctor, learn about any possible side effects, and then decide which (if any) medication is right for you. Our ethos is not to push for or against medication, as we recognise that people can get better with or without, provided they undertake the kind of work we suggest in this book.

## DEPRESSION – SUMMARY

- It is common to have a depressive illness alongside body image problems and BDD.
- Treatment for depression can include anti-depressant medication and a course of CBT therapy.
- When you are depressed it is hard to motivate yourself to do things, so a **behaviour booster** is the first step in overcoming a depressive episode.
- Using strategies to challenge unhelpful thinking is also very useful, including using the Two Hands Technique, and identifying and changing any thinking problems.

# SECTION 15

# COSMETIC PROCEDURES

Some people with BDD or body image issues consider cosmetic procedures as a way of changing their appearance and helping them feel better about themselves. The belief is that, if you're unhappy with your appearance, then anything you can do to physically change your appearance at least offers hope that you will feel better. Therefore, it must be a good thing. However, research shows that most people with a significant body image issue or BDD are usually dissatisfied with the outcome of surgery.[21] For some people surgery can actually worsen their concerns about their appearance. For others, satisfaction with the outcome of surgery wears off over time.

Why is this the case? The answer lies in our understanding of what the problem is, and what the problem isn't. The problem with a body image issue or BDD is how someone feels about and experiences their appearance; it is not a problem with their appearance or a particular feature. So, what they really want is to not be consumed by this worry and feel better about their appearance – they assume that an altered appearance can provide this. In short, it doesn't!

Instead, this is something that we can achieve with a good psychological intervention – such as this book – without resorting to surgery.

## GOALS FOR SURGERY

In the case where there is not an objectively noticeable flaw with their appearance, it can be very difficult for the patient and surgeon to agree on what cosmetic procedure is required. For example, Richard was unhappy with his ears, but wasn't adequately able to explain why. He didn't think they were too big, or too small; he just knew they didn't look 'right'. His friends couldn't see the problem, but this didn't discourage Richard from feeling like he needed surgery. Of course, as his expectations of surgery were vague and hard to define, it is then difficult for him to assess whether or not the operation will be successful and whether the risks that are inherent in any surgery were worth the potential gains. In this case, the surgeon agreed with Richard that he would first undertake a course of CBT to focus on improving his body image and self-confidence. Afterwards, if he still wanted surgery on his ears, they could discuss the possibility again.

Others can pinpoint exactly what feature they would like to be altered. They have researched it extensively, and want to specify to the surgeon exactly what surgery is required for their desired outcome. However, as significant body image issues and BDD can fluctuate, so does someone's experience of their perceived flaw. There can be times when it feels less of an issue and less obvious, and there can be times when it feels as though it is the most significant feature about that person (we have discussed this previously as emotional reasoning). Their view is based on what they feel, not what is objective. You can see how this would make it tricky to explain what they want changed in surgery as their feelings about their appearance fluctuate.

## EXPECTATIONS

Then there is the issue of expectations of outcome of the surgery. Before surgery, people can have a range of expectations of what a successful surgery could provide them with. In people with body image issues and BDD, this is rarely simply an aesthetic one. They have an expectation of the difference in appearance, but they will also expect their feelings to change. They might also have expectations about what these new feelings may allow them to do that they have previously been struggling with. Expectations can include hopes of improved confidence, being more attractive to other people, being more successful, being able to go out more, being able to feel normal and less self-conscious. A cosmetic intervention cannot fulfil all the additional expectations associated with the appearance change.

## OUTCOME

Following surgery, people with body image issues or BDD usually respond in a couple of ways:

- They feel that the surgery has been moderately successful, but wish the surgeon had altered things "just a bit more", and therefore they seek further surgery.
- They are not happy with the outcome as they can't 'feel' or "see" a noticeable difference.
- They think they have made things worse by the alteration, and want to change it back to how it looked before.

- They think the results are too obvious, and as a consequence feel like people are now looking at them because of the change in their appearance.
- They are happy with the outcome but this change highlights other areas that now appear odd to them. They then seek to alter those too.

These typical reactions show that gauging the success of cosmetic surgery is never straightforward. These outcomes can often lead to further body dissatisfaction, not the improved self-image that people would be hoping for. That is because, unfortunately, there isn't any reliable evidence showing that cosmetic surgery leads to psychological wellbeing for people with BDD or body image problems.[22]

We often see that even in cases where someone with BDD or body image issues is initially satisfied with the results of surgery, the level of satisfaction doesn't last. Sometimes they become fixated on a different area of their body instead and may seek further surgery for that area after a period of preoccupation.

However, realistically, we know that many people consider cosmetic surgery. What we recommend is that before you take steps down this route, you consider that surgery may not actually 'fix' the problem and improve your self-confidence or your relationship with your body. Surgery may just be another, rather extreme, safety behaviour and one that can be difficult to undo. So before you explore cosmetic surgery as an option, we strongly advise that you undertake a course of treatment to improve your body image and BDD and address your expectations of surgery. Then, following this treatment, you can assess again how necessary you believe surgery is.

So if surgery is something that you are considering, please ask yourself:

- Do I have a clear idea of what it is I would like to be physically altered?
- What are my expectations of the surgery?
- Do I hope that I will feel differently about myself after the surgery?
- Do I hope that others will respond differently to me after the surgery?
- After the surgery do I think that I will be able to do things that I currently struggle to do?
- How will I know if surgery has been "successful"?
- Will success depend on whether the feature is smaller / larger straighter / more symmetrical, or will it mostly be based on how I feel about myself and my appearance?

If your answers are predominantly about how differently you will feel because of your hopes that you have an altered or changed appearance, you would probably benefit from working on your body image and expectations first, before undergoing cosmetic surgery.

We would suggest discussing your expectations honestly with your surgeon. Good surgeons will not perform an operation until they are satisfied that you are likely to have the outcome you hope for. If they believe that you have serious body image issues or BDD, they will encourage you to seek psychological help first before even considering surgery. Most cosmetic surgeons just want the best outcome for their patients – whether it is a surgical outcome, or improving their psychological wellbeing and relationship with their body – or both.

## SURGERY – SUMMARY

- It is common for people with body image issues and BDD to seek cosmetic surgery or other procedures to try and 'fix' their perceived flaw or features.

- Body image and BDD is a problem with how we feel and experience our body and appearance, it is not a problem with our actual appearance.

- Our body image can fluctuate which can affect our desire for surgery, and the expectations we have for the outcome.

- Surgery will not change other things in your life, such as relationships, work, and your emotional state, nor is it guaranteed to improve your body image or self confidence.

- Cosmetic surgery for people with significant body image concerns or BDD is not recommended and typically predicts a dissatisfied outcome which can actually make the problem worse.

- It is important to have clear expectations for the outcome of surgery.

- Talk about your expectations for surgery honestly with the surgeon; they will help guide you on the best course of action.

# SECTION 16

# KEEPING WELL

Now that you've come so far and made so much progress, we need to consider two things:

- How do you stay well?
- What do you do if you feel yourself slipping?

In this chapter we'll help you draw up a blueprint for staying well, and for dealing with any body image problems if they re-emerge.

The first thing we want you to do is think about what you've already achieved, because now you need to try to maintain your new, more positive attitude towards yourself and your body.

Of course, we all know that nothing is stable in life. Any one of us can have a bad day, and any one of us can experience things that shake our confidence. So it's unreasonable to expect that you will go through life without the occasional setback. But always remember – if you do have a setback, it doesn't mean that you're going to go back to how you were before.

Here's an example: I (Lauren) have a knee injury that I got from running. Now, as long as I carry on running and look after myself, the knee generally feels okay. I have to make sure I stretch and keep the muscles strong and supple. If I notice a twinge, then I know I need to put some ice on it and go back to my physio stretches to stop it from getting worse. There is still the chance it might flare up, but I'm okay with that, because I know what my treatment plan is. I might need to go back for a couple of sessions of physiotherapy. I might need to try some different exercises to strengthen my quads and gently stretch my hamstrings, and I'll probably need to rest it for a little while. But if I do all of that, then I know the symptoms will abate quite quickly. If I don't look after myself and continue running, it will flare up and become a much bigger problem.

It's the same for you. We hope that you're going to stay well. But you have the reassurance of knowing that if the body image issues or BDD flare up again, you have all the tools you need in this book to take control again. Just like Chloe has been able to do. She has had a few flare ups, and in each case, she has been able to deal with it.

The way you think about what's happening to you is important too. If things get hard, don't think of it as a relapse, think of it as a 'blip' or a 'temporary setback'. And remember that you have responded well to the techniques we've outlined for you in this book, so you can do it again. And this time, the likelihood is that the process will be that much quicker.

## WHAT DO YOU DO IF YOU START TO WORRY ABOUT SOMETHING ELSE?

Let's think about what you need to do if, the next time you have a body image issue, it's about something different, i.e. a different body part or feature to any you have worried about before ...

You might think it means that you have an entirely new issue about your appearance, rather than a different manifestation of your worry problem. But it is almost certainly going to be a continuation of your worry problem about your appearance – having had it before, it is more likely that it will happen again. If the things you are worrying about now are different to the things you worried about before, don't worry. The same strategies will still apply.

Here are some questions to help you build up your own plan to stay well and overcome any blip. We have included a copy of Chloe's staying well plan to help you.

---

**What were your worries before?**
Mainly that my neck stuck out and there were visible hairs all over my face and arms.

**What were your triggers?**
Seeing other people
Looking in a mirror
Taking showers and getting changed
Touching my neck

---

**What is your new way of thinking about yourself now?**

*I know it is a worry problem – I was worrying too much about my appearance, and what other people think about me. I am not wholly defined by my appearance, and there are many more interesting things and qualities that define me.*

How do you see yourself as a person?

*I am a good person. People tell me I'm kind, and although I sometimes lack confidence, I know that I am a good friend, sister and daughter – and also that I write well.*

What things did you find most helpful in this book?

*The thinking error exercises*

*Ways to stop rumination*

*And the experiments! Even though they were really hard, they made the most difference to my life!*

What were your worries before?

What were your triggers?

**What is your new way of thinking about yourself now?**

**How do you see yourself as a person?**
(Not just in terms of your appearance.)

**What things did you find most helpful in this book?**

## LOOKING AHEAD, WHAT DO YOU NEED TO WATCH OUT FOR?

You need to be aware of the things that might trigger worries like these in future. These might include a comment from somebody, a worry about a new area of your body, weight changes, relationship issues, or a change in circumstances that means you can't exercise or do your hobbies etc.

**I need to watch out for:**

What things can I do if I notice I am becoming preoccupied again?

- Start monitoring your thoughts and challenging them as they arise and come up with new ways of thinking about yourself.

- Carry on doing exposure experiments.

- Talk to someone supportive – for example a friend or family member, or someone who'll be able to encourage you.

- You may need to consider going back on medication.

-

-

-

-

## KEEPING WELL – SUMMARY

- Having a plan can help us stay well and deal with setbacks.

- Setbacks or blips are normal, and are not the same as relapses. If they happen, it is important to start using the techniques you have learnt to overcome them quickly.

- If your worry starts again, focusing on a new feature or aspect of your appearance, you can still use all the same strategies you have covered in this book to overcome it.

## SECTION 17

## LIFE AFTER BDD

As you now know, my life has improved so much since meeting Lauren and Annemarie. There's more that I'd like to achieve, though, and there's no reason to believe I can't do it, with my new tools in place to help me. So, looking even further ahead, I'd like to work towards being independent and living by myself. I'd like regular, steady work five days a week and a normal routine – getting up every day and doing something constructive. That's important to me and I think that learning to depend on yourself is a big part of recovery.

The fact that I'm even thinking like this shows that I've made significant progress. Sometimes, when I look back, I can't believe just how far I've come. Today, I am doing what I want to do. I have left my part-time job and I am following my passion. I'm a freelance writer, and I review films. Just saying that sounds unbelievable! How did I get from feeling suicidal to doing the one thing I have always wanted to do?

With Lauren and Annemarie's help, I have learnt how to find some peace. I don't run from my feelings – I embrace them. The strength that I've found has helped me to start turning my life around. Two years ago, I could not have done this. I couldn't even have imagined doing it. Even one year ago, I wouldn't have been ready. But things have changed so much.

I don't live a life without depression, but I know how to live with it. And BDD no longer rules my life. And now, at last, I am working towards being the person I want to be. I understand that, even when I don't feel great, I can get through almost anything.

The uncertainty of earning a living is scary. But life is full of uncertainties. I'm still in the process of establishing regular income. Right now I just have a bit of money coming in here and there, but I knew I needed to take the plunge and leave my retail job. I knew that I was finally in the right headspace to do it. That's thanks to the work we've done over the last couple of years.

I know that my parents are very proud of me. My sense of independence has truly soared, thanks in no small part to their encouragement and support. They understand there are good and bad days, but all the small victories add up and we try to reflect on this during tougher times. It's definitely brought us closer.

Sometimes I catastrophise my situation when I worry that my writing's not good enough and I'm not going to make enough money. I know freelance writing is a fickle field and sometimes worry about where I will be in the future. But Lauren told me to break every goal down into smaller goals. Where do I see myself in three or six months' time? Rather than worrying where I will be in five years, I know can do some great things in that time. I've just passed my driving theory exam, for example. That's a huge step for me.

I am getting better at breaking my goals and my worries down into smaller chunks and addressing them bit by bit. When you've dealt with such dark feelings of depression, you can put the uncertainty of daily life into perspective. I'm not hugely confident yet, but I know that I have the ability in me to do good work. Maybe one day I can even speak at the annual BDD Foundation Conference – just considering that idea a year or two ago would have terrified me, but now, it's certainly something I'd like to do.

I'd like to help the people who are experiencing what I have experienced. One of the first things I wrote after going freelance was a column on BDD for the Geeks Vs Loneliness section of the Den of Geek website. I opened up about my life with BDD, and I didn't hold back. I told readers about the tsunami of self-hate that assailed me when I caught a glimpse of my reflection. I told them about my dread of school photo day, about my deteriorating social life and how I spent years a virtual prisoner in my own bedroom. I revealed everything about my camouflaging techniques and my automatic assumptions that everyone I met hated me. It was the first time I had been so public about my own BDD. I was honest and it felt good to open up and reach out to others.

Of course I was apprehensive about doing it, because I knew how easy it is for people hiding behind a computer screen to leave hurtful comments. But my goal for writing the article was simple: I felt that if it helped even one person, then it would all be worth it. So I was delighted when I got such an outpouring of support and comments. People shared their stories about body image and body dissatisfaction. It was wonderful to see so much more attention being given to this still little-known topic. I thought about how I would have felt reading this just a few years ago, and how it might just have helped to know that crucial truth: you are not alone.

I wish I had known that when I was growing up. In those dark times when I was curled up on my bedroom floor weeping to the song 'Out There' from The Hunchback of Notre Dame, I never knew there was anyone else who thought like I did. My diagnosis changed things. It would have been far better if I was diagnosed earlier. But the diagnosis wasn't enough on its own anyway; it was the intervention from Lauren and Annemarie that really started to turn my life around.

Now, I know that everyone has some sort of concerns about their body image, but I only really had my lightbulb moment when I had the specialist knowledge that they gave me. CBT was so general when I was first introduced to it, so having their in-depth understanding of CBT as it relates to body image really made a difference. When I met Lauren and then Annemarie I immediately felt like they understood. Body dysmorphia is such a delicate issue that you really need to work with people who specialise in the area. And their approach was so important in helping me address my BDD. I dread to think where I'd be without them.

If you're struggling, try to find a support network that suits you. For me, the BDD Foundation[23] was a real lifeline. I have been to both of their annual BDD conferences and I really recommend them – not just as a resource for finding out more, but as a way of reminding people that they are not alone. I love hearing the individual speakers, and it can feel quite profound when someone says something that really hits home with your own experience of BDD.

One of the girls I saw at the last annual BDD Foundation conference had been involved in a TV programme in which she'd had her photos taken professionally. So I watched the programme with Mum and Dad and everything she said really hit home. I was trying hard not to cry because it was just so **me**. After she'd had her photo taken, everyone was saying how nice it was, and her sister couldn't understand why she was so upset because she was so beautiful. But the girl was looking at the photos and seeing all the imperfections. Even though I couldn't see the imperfections she was seeing, I could really empathise with her. I understood.

Hearing other peoples' stories has really helped me. Even when I first saw Lauren, and I knew she had dealt with patients with BDD and body image issues, I still didn't know anyone else who had it. So I did a lot of searching online, and found some useful documentaries on YouTube. For me, anything that made my BDD more relatable was useful, and getting other people's views on their experiences of BDD really helped. Knowing how much value I got from their stories really inspired me to write my own.

I'm not embarrassed by my BDD any more. And I think people generally are getting more used to BDD as a concept. The more people who know about it, and are aware of it, the better. So I think it's so important that we talk openly about BDD and body image issues.

The starting point – something that would have really helped me – is school. Children are attributing their self-worth to their image in primary school now. I'm worried that we will start to see cases of BDD and body image problems in nine and ten year olds soon if we're not careful. So we should have positive, open discussion on body image and introduce positive body image classes as part of a national curriculum subject in our schools. If I had been more aware of body image when I was younger, maybe my BDD wouldn't have got to the point it got to. It might not have lasted as long, or been as severe. Maybe I would also have had a diagnosis quicker.

So, we really do need to educate ourselves more. The media always want to make a story out of conditions like this. I think there definitely should be better media guidelines for something as important and sensitive as mental health – they shouldn't put a spin on it. They should just present the facts, rather than sensationalising it into a story. They shouldn't make it sound like we're just the self-obsessed generation that takes too many selfies. Everyone loves to point the finger, but they're less eager to listen. That's how you come about general ignorance and comments on media stories such as 'Don't you just think this is what all teenagers go through? They're just being a bit vain.'

I think we also need better screening of people who go for cosmetic surgery, to be able to identify those who are suffering with BDD and get them the appropriate care without them having to go through invasive medical procedures.

In terms of treatment, the rule for BDD should be "the earlier, the better". Specialist care also needs to be made more easily available. We need more research into the condition, and more therapists specialising in BDD and body image issues. I've been very fortunate to have the care I've had.

In Part I, I asked if I would ever recover from BDD …

It has been a long journey and I am still working my way towards a new life for myself, but I can tell you that I think completely differently about my body dysmorphia now.

It hasn't always been easy. For me, one of the most difficult stages – and this might go for you too – was when I had to start dropping my safety behaviours.

It wasn't just difficult; it was actually scary! My brain was almost split in two over which interpretation from the Two Hands Thinking Technique was correct. It was like a tug of war. My irrational side had been in control for so long that, at first, I found it hard to correct the balance. Every now and then I can still feel that paranoid part of me emerging, but at least now I know how to deal with it so much better.

So for example, I mentioned that the hair on my arms had always been a great concern for me. I hated how dark and thick it was. That's why I used to shave my arms to try to avoid anyone from seeing it and judging me for it. But I let the hair on my forearm keep growing, so I could put myself to the test.

My old thinking had made me believe that the hair was the problem. But Annemarie encouraged me to test that theory out. I wore a short-sleeved t-shirt and went out in public, fearing the worst. But no one said anything to me. I wasn't even aware of anyone looking at my arms at all. People weren't judging me. My problem really was my worry about the hair on my arms, not the hair itself.

So, just like I had learnt to go out in public without wearing a scarf, I learnt to go out wearing whatever I wanted to wear. And that's because the evidence kept stacking up to show me that people were not looking and making negative judgments about my appearance, like my old worries had me believe.

I still have concerns, and I have lived with my old way of thinking for so long that some old habits die hard. So, for example, I can leave the house without a mirror, but if I'm feeling a bit vulnerable, I will still have to be careful not to catch my reflection in a shop window, because seeing myself from an obscure angle or in weird lighting can make my unhelpful thoughts spiral. But at least if that happens, I know I can combat my negative thoughts.

I know what situations cause my BDD to flare up, and in some cases, these situations can't be avoided. But it only really happens a couple of times a month – at most – and I'm far more equipped to tackle my responses. Of course, it still takes a lot of effort. But I can tell you that, the more you practise the new ways of thinking and interpreting events, the easier it becomes. I have made them a habit so that they get more and more intuitive. I'm working towards the day when I can change or ignore any negative image thought the moment it springs up. That's my ultimate goal.

Of course, my journey has had many downs as well as ups. In Part II I talked about how the first time I tried exposure therapy, it didn't work the way that I hoped. Perhaps you have had a bad experience of therapy too. If you have, I would say that although it just compounds the horrible worry that you can't get better, my advice would be to reflect on the experience you've had and use what you learn to help you decide on the qualities and experience you're looking for in a therapist.

If you are going to be working with a therapist – and if you're going to get the most out of the experience – you need to be absolutely at ease with them. And they need to know what they are doing! Be honest with yourself and don't be afraid to try other options. It can be a lengthy process but once you find the right fit, it will be a therapeutic union that can turn your life around. And I feel like I have turned my life around now.

I really hope that reading this book is the turning point for you, just like meeting Lauren and Annemarie was the turning point for me. Although your journey will be different to mine, I know that the techniques they reveal in this book will help you make so much progress. They helped me in so many ways – and I think it's so wonderful that all the exercises and experiments that helped me so much are all in this book so that they can help you too.

Even if things get difficult, please, stay with it. You can do it and you will be so pleased that you did! Good luck with your journey.

# SECTION 18

# A MOTHER'S PERSPECTIVE

If you're the parent of a child with body image issues or BDD, you want to do everything you can to help your son or daughter. While I know that my experience of living with my daughter's BDD will be different to your experience, I'm sure your son or daughter can get better. And this book will really help you both.

There may be times when you feel alone, or perhaps you worry that there was something you could have done to help your child earlier. But BDD isn't like that – it sneaks up on you. For a while I didn't notice that there was anything particularly wrong with Chloe. And you might not notice it with your son or daughter. But you shouldn't blame yourself for that. Nowadays, most teens have problems with their appearance and self-esteem. So, although she said things which might have rung alarm bells in retrospect, it didn't seem unusual at first.

The time I really started noticing that something was wrong was when she went to Alton Towers when she was 16. (She talks about it in Chapter 2.) She was having a hard time anyway because her grandfather, my father, had just taken a fall and it wasn't long after her grandmother, my mother, had passed away. It was a really difficult trip for her, and afterwards, she told me that she was desperately unhappy. She said she hated how she looked, and hated that her friends were putting pictures of her up on social media. She made it sound like they were doing it to tease her.

From the outside looking in, BDD doesn't seem to make sense. It's really strange when you look at Chloe and her twin sister together and see how similar they look. In fact, they're pretty much the same in terms of appearance. And yet, Chloe didn't see anything wrong in the way Olivia looked and that made it seem even more challenging and confusing than it might otherwise have been.

Of course, we didn't know about BDD then. And to begin with, the most difficult thing was encouraging Chloe to acknowledge that she had a problem, so that she could get help for it. Before we knew it was BDD I thought it was just a depressive condition. I thought a big part of it was the grief brought on by my parents' deaths.

In 2010 she agreed to see a doctor and got the first round of counselling, but it didn't really help. What did help was getting that first diagnosis of Body Dysmorphic Disorder in 2012. After that, I was able to do some research and found that she ticked almost all the boxes when it came to her behaviour and symptoms. We then had a little bit more of an understanding of what was going on.

The question there, then, was 'Who do we go to for help?' There was no specialist support available in Sussex. We had to go further afield. So I did a lot of research and it soon became obvious that one of the leading specialists in the field was Professor Veale. We spoke to Chloe's GP who, happily, sent us a referral to Professor Veale. He was then able to give us an official diagnosis of BDD. Getting that diagnosis helped make sense of a lot of things, but of course, it was just the start.

Acceptance of mental health issues still has a long way to go, but it is improving. At the time of Chloe's diagnosis though, there was still a real stigma about mental health issues and we didn't want to force her to talk about it if she didn't want to. However, things did become easier when she felt she was able to acknowledge her illness publicly, especially in terms of explaining things if she couldn't turn up to an event.

It was difficult, and it was upsetting. And it's a shame to know that one day we'll look back on these types of things and feel sad that she wasn't there to enjoy it with us. They are times that we'll never get back. But what I need Chloe to know, and what I think it would be good for all friends or family members of someone suffering with BDD to convey, is that I know it's nothing personal. It's not a wilful or spiteful act, it's just an unfortunate consequence of her condition.

After the diagnosis, it did enable Chloe to be a bit more vocal about the specific parts of her body she disliked, such as her neck and the pores on her face, although really she hated every part of herself.

Even before she started seeing Lauren and Annemarie, Chloe found that talking to her first BDD therapist was a big help because she finally felt as though she was discussing it with someone who really knew what she was going through. And she really needed that. After that, the biggest and most positive step forward was when she met Lauren and Annemarie and started therapy with them.

I didn't find it too difficult talking to close friends about it. I was lucky that a lot of them had health and social care backgrounds and they were very supportive. I myself work for Care and Support West Sussex, and so I meet a lot of carers, support carers, and young carers who have worked with people with mental illnesses – people who understood the situation. But I think that even if you don't know anyone who necessarily understands what BDD is straightaway, awareness is growing. Talking to someone can really help. Because as you'll know, there are times when it is really hard.

For me, one of the most difficult things was knowing that there wasn't anything I could say or do to help. Obviously, it's not like it's something very visual or easily fixable like a scraped knee. I couldn't just give her a hug and a kiss and make everything okay. That part is particularly hard for a parent or a carer. And it was especially hard for me because I am the type that likes solving problems and finding solutions to things. There was no immediate or easy solution to this.

Supportive words become meaningless and not very effective when you're dealing with a deeply ingrained mental illness, too. If I ever told Chloe she looked nice, she would say, 'You would say that. You're my mother.' Words are just words and they didn't help. It was hard to stop the feelings of guilt. I doubted myself and questioned myself so much. I thought I must have missed something when Chloe was growing up – if only I could have spotted it happening and stopped it in its tracks.

But you worry about every aspect of the BDD. It is so stressful on everyone – and there are times when it feels like you're walking on eggshells, when you're worried about what will happen next and if it's going to be another setback.

It also made us worry about the future. We only ever wanted the best for Chloe, but we knew that her BDD limited her options. Though we tried to support her through her exams and education, I think I knew deep down, in my heart, that she wouldn't be able to go through with a lot of it. It became clear that she just wasn't able to focus. And while we always encouraged her to reach her potential, we never had any concerns of her letting us down. We love her and we only ever wanted her to be as happy as she could be.

There were times when her progress seemed to stall, and during those times it was hard to remind ourselves that she was still moving forward. It was an emotional rollercoaster. There were times when we wanted to talk about Chloe's BDD as a family, but we always waited until she was ready. Sometimes she felt okay enough to talk to us about it, but we knew it was important for Chloe to have her private space. Occasionally she talked about her therapy, but she didn't go into lots of detail. Other than that, therapy was quite a private affair for her.

Things haven't been easy for any of us. You may well have found this too – even though you **know** your loved one is suffering from BDD or body image problems, it can still be very hard to understand, unless you have experienced BDD or body image issues yourself. So it can be frustrating for everyone. My husband is a scientist and is very logical by nature, so it's always been a struggle for him; he looks at Chloe and sees no significant physical difference or abnormality. And obviously, it's not easy because Olivia and Chloe are identical.

I found it really helpful to read up on as much information as I could. Professors Veale's presentation at the BDD conference really helped us too, and helped us visualise things more easily.

It's really important that you have your own coping strategies too. So, if I ever need some time out, I know what I need to do and I know how to look after myself. Daily therapy for myself is taking the dog for a walk, or reading a magazine. My own health and wellbeing is important, so that I can look after my daughter.

I also think it's really important for Chloe to do things for herself. It's always better if she makes her own doctor's appointment, or gets her own prescription, so we have always encouraged her to take as much autonomy over her recovery as possible.

It's still nice when we're all together as a family, and my husband and Olivia are very supportive. Olivia works for the NHS and my husband works in the health service too, so they have the right kind of knowledge that allows them to be supportive.

We have good things to look forward to. Olivia is getting married and Chloe is going to be a bridesmaid, so I really hope we can all enjoy that. I know it won't be easy for her, but I think she'll get through it okay. She's preparing for it with Annemarie. Any event in the public domain will be more challenging for Chloe than it would be for others. And we all need to remember that what seems like an ordinary event to us can be so much harder for someone with BDD or body image issues.

I'm proud that Chloe has worked so hard – not just on this book – but throughout her recovery from BDD. She's definitely come a long way. Before, she couldn't go out without make-up and lots of layers on to hide her neck. She wouldn't leave the house alone either. Now, she'll willingly go shopping alone, with no make-up on. She will go to London by herself to see film screenings for her freelance film critic job. She still struggles a bit in large groups, but she's getting there.

She still needs to develop a bit more self-belief. She wants a good career, and I know that she's smart enough and talented enough to do whatever she wants to do, but that confidence has to come from within. She's insightful and thinks things through a lot, but she just needs to find that balance between thinking things through logically and overthinking. Overall, though, she's improved massively. And I look forward to the time that Chloe can live her life 100% to the fullest, and have more confidence in herself.

I know how hard it is when you want to support someone you love as they struggle with BDD or body image issues. My advice is to do as much research and reading as you can. Learn about other people who have the condition, those who are at different places on the severity spectrum. It helps you realise that you're not alone.

I would also say that you need to remember that as relatives or friends, we can provide as much support as we're willing to give, but fixing the problem comes from the sufferer themselves. Only they can make that decision to help themselves. There is no silver bullet or magic wand. It will take hard work to find a solution.

In terms of dealing with things yourself, remember that it will be an emotional rollercoaster. There will be ups and downs and it's okay for you to have these feelings sometimes. I try hard not to express frustration, but it's not always that easy. Sometimes when things go wrong or if Chloe is having a bad day, it's easy to think, 'Oh no, it's happening again.' But it's an illness, and it needs to be managed, and it's okay to have bad days sometimes.

If you can, and if you want to, I think it's really beneficial to keep trying to raise the profile of this illness. Diagnosis is becoming more prevalent, but we're still 10–15 years behind eating disorders in terms of social awareness. There is still a long way to go and we need all the help we can get in raising awareness. Good luck to you.

 ***Lauren and Annemarie:*** It can be hard to know what to expect when your friend or loved one has body image issues or BDD. Equally, knowing what to do and say can be hard when your friend or loved one is clearly distressed by their problems. And as Chloe's mother has said, it can be very frustrating watching someone you care about criticise their appearance and doubt themselves so much, when you think there is nothing wrong with the way they look!

Hopefully by reading this book you will get a greater understanding of how difficult – or rather, impossible – it is for people with body image issues and BDD to be objective about themselves. So please have a little patience with them.

When people decide to tackle their body image issues or BDD, it is a very brave step and they can really benefit from your support. However, the key thing to bear in mind is that it is a process, and that means that their recovery will take some time (some people will find the recovery process easier and quicker than others). Treatment and recovery will not always be a neat and tidy process with a clearly defined end point. Knowing that they will have ups and downs can help keep your expectations realistic. But it can also help take the pressure off your friend or loved one, so that they know they can confide in you if they're having a bad day.

Whatever their experience is, it's important to know that you can play an important part in helping them work through this process. Here are some of the key things you can do to help:

- **Be prepared for setbacks.** The path your friend or loved one is taking is a difficult one. There will be times when they feel less able to cope with the process, and at those times you can encourage them, in a positive way, to keep going.

- **Be yourself.** One of the things people value most about the support of friends and loved ones is their unique perspective, and sense of humour. It will really help to reduce their stress (and yours) if you both keep a positive sense of humour and can have a laugh together.

- **Try to not blame the person with body image problems or BDD.** It's not their fault and they certainly don't want to have these problems.

- **Try not to problem-solve the issue for them.** Examples include finding new skin products, paying for dermatological interventions, making excuses for them not going to events, or for missing work or school etc. These things only reinforce the person's belief that there is something wrong with the way they look and that it needs to be changed. That only takes away the responsibility they have to help themselves.

- **Set clear boundaries at home.** If the person's problems are impacting on their home life, e.g. they're taking too long in the bathroom and making other people late for school or work, it's helpful to set clear boundaries at home, like setting time limits in the bathroom in the morning.

- **Appreciate that they'll be uncomfortable from time to time.** As a friend or family member, you will inevitably want to ease their discomfort, but you need to appreciate that they'll face discomfort (such as anxiety as part of their recovery. For example, if they tell you that their habituation exercises are difficult, it's important that you remain positive about the experience they're going through and try to encourage them to keep going.

- **Try not to answer their requests for reassurance.**
  Although it's very hard, please don't answer your loved
  one's questions when they try to check how they're
  looking. This is giving reassurance, which is actually
  part of the problem, as we discussed in Part I, Chapter
  2. While it's normal to reassure the people we love,
  reassurance can turn into a type of 'fix', and it will never
  be enough to help. It can be a good idea to practise a
  few compassionate statements that you can use
  instead of giving reassurance. For example, 'It's not
  helpful for me to tell you that … (you look okay, etc
  Can I do something else to help you get ready tonight?
  Perhaps give you a lift?' Or, 'I know you're feeling
  anxious about things, what can you do, or what can we
  do, to help you get through this right now?'

- **Know that you cannot make someone better or
  more optimistic.** There is a limit to what any of us can
  do. However, you can always give encouragement, urge
  them to stick with their treatment programme, or
  suggest they see a doctor if they need additional help
  or support.

- **Look after yourself!** As Chloe's mother said it can be
  very difficult and frustrating watching someone you
  love battle through body image problems or BDD, but
  in order to remain positive and give support, you also
  need to be mentally healthy and secure. So make sure
  you have some time for yourself and enjoy some stress
  relieving activities.

- **Read this book!** It can be really useful for your friend
  or loved one to know that there is somebody else who

understands the treatment path they're on. When you read the book and you'll be able to give them even more support.

And finally, if you are really concerned about your loved one's health and wellbeing, **please go and speak to your local doctor or a mental health team**. It may feel like you are "betraying" the person you love, but you want them to get better, and sometimes we need to bring in external help for that to happen.

# CONCLUSION

 ***Lauren and Annemarie:*** Congratulations for sticking with the programme and getting to this point. The approach we've described in this book is based on sound clinical principles and years of psychological research. It is suitable for anyone suffering with BDD and body image issues. Best of all, as we hope we have shown, it is easy to understand and the techniques are easy to learn. The difficulty is having the courage to face your body image problems and BDD – but you have taken the first step by working through this book. Now, it is up to you to continue the great work that you've started.

Hopefully you now have the confidence – as well as the techniques – to change your life, just like Chloe has. There may well be times when the journey still feels difficult, but as long as you remember everything we've talked about and apply it to your life, you will be able to move towards a life that is not dominated by BDD and body image issues. You will be able to move on and experience a whole new way of life.

Chloe now has so much more freedom to do the things that she wants to do. More than that, she is a stronger person. As she continues her way in the world, she may find that she is more resilient for having had – and overcome – mental health issues. She has shown strength, perseverance, and an incredible determination to succeed.

Remember to refer back to this book whenever you need to. It is your manual for overcoming your body image issues and BDD. It is a way to kick-start a more fulfilling life for yourself.

You have seen that your body image issues and BDD, as well as the anxiety and stress you feel about your body, are inspired by various triggers. It is the trigger that sets off the spiral of cognitive, emotional, physiological and physical symptoms you feel. But now you know that by changing the way you interpret these triggers, tolerating your emotions, and challenging your behaviours, you can change the cycle and build a better and more caring relationship with yourself and your body.

If you have the courage to embark on this journey, you will never look back. Do please remember to treat yourself kindly along the way. We appreciate that this isn't always easy. When things are difficult, or you don't feel as if you are making quite as much progress as you would like, it is easy to blame yourself. But never forget, your body image issues are not your fault, nor are they a sign of weakness. Just like a physical injury such as a broken leg, the healing process works better if you accept it and follow the right treatment plan. You can't simply stop your leg from being broken in the first place, or beat yourself up for having a broken leg.

We hope you have embraced the journey we've shared with you in this book, and that you have found the inspiration and the tools you need to beat your body image issues and start a new life for yourself.

We wish you every success on your journey.

# REFERENCES

1 Gilbert, P. (2010). *The Compassionate Mind: A New Approach to Life's Challenge.* Oakland, CA: New Harbinger Publications.

2 Rosen, J.C., Reiter, J., Orosan, P., Veale, D., and Williams (1995). *Cognitive-]behavioural body image therapy for body dysmorphic disorder.* Journal of Consulting and Clinical Psychology, 63(2), 263–69.

Veale, D., Gournay, K., Dryden, W., Boocock, A., Shah, F., Willson, R., and Walburn, J. (1996). *Body dysmorphic disorder: A cognitive behavioural model and pilot randomized controlled trial.* Behaviour Research and Therapy, 34(9), 717–29.

3 American Psychiatric Association. (2013). *Diagnostic and Statistical Manual of Mental Disorders* (5th ed.). Washington, DC: American Psychiatric Association.

4 Amsterdam, B. (1972). *Mirror self-image reactions before age two.* Developmental Psychology, 5, 297–305.

Anderson, J. R. (1984). *The development of self-recognition: A review.* Developmental Psychobiology, 17, 35–49.

Neisser, U. (1993). *The perceived self.* New York: Cambridge University Press.

5 Merton, R. K. (1948). *The self-fulfilling prophecy.* Antioch Review, 8, 193–210.

6 Veale and Neziroglu et al. (2008). *The self in understanding and treating psychological disorders*, 126.

7 American Psychiatric Association. (2013). *Diagnostic and Statistical Manual of Mental Disorders* (5th ed.). Washington, DC: American Psychiatric Association.

8 Ibid.

9 Ibid.

10 Ibid.

11 Ibid.

12 Ibid.

13 Ibid.

14 Ibid.

15 Beck, J. S. (2011). *Cognitive Behavior Therapy: Basics and Beyond* (2nd ed). New York: Guilford.

16 Ibid.

17 NICE. (2005). *Obsessive-compulsive disorder and body dysmorphic disorder: treatment*. Retrieved from www.nice.org.uk/guidance/cg31.

18 American Psychiatric Association. (2013). *Diagnostic and Statistical Manual of Mental Disorders* (5th ed.). Washington, DC: American Psychiatric Association.

19 Ibid.

20 Dimidjian, S., Hollon, S. D., Dobson, K. S., Schmaling, K. B., Kohlenberg, R. J., Addis, M. E., and Atkins, D. C. (2006). *Randomized trial of behavioral activation, cognitive therapy, and antidepressant medication in the acute treatment of adults with major depression*. Journal of Consulting and Clinical Psychology, 74(4), 658.

21 NICE guidelines.

22 Crerand, C. E., Phillips, K. A., Menard, W., & Fay, C. (2005). Nonpsychiatric medical treatment of body dysmorphic disorder. Psychosomatics, 46, 549–55.

Phillips, K. A., Grant, J., Siniscalchi, J., & Albertini, R. S. (2001). *Surgical and nonpsychiatric medical treatment of patients with body dysmorphic disorder*. Psychosomatics, 42, 504–10.

23 Crerand, C. E., Menard, W., & Phillips, K. A. (2010). *Surgical and minimally invasive cosmetic procedures among persons with body dysmorphic disorder*. Annals of Plastic Surgery, 65, 11–16.

24 The BDD Foundation is a UK charity with a global reach. You can find out more at: www.bddfoundation.org

# INDEX

## A

abnormality 347

achievement 130, 308–10, 313;
  and enjoyment effort 314;
  sense of 308–10, 313

acne 65

activities 22, 30, 136-8, 193–4, 288, 307, 309–14;
  favourite 311;
  half-term 31;
  manageable 124;
  physical 99;
  pleasurable 304;
  preferred 193

adolescence 99, 102

adrenaline
  anxiety-fueled 21;
  surges 21–2, 97

age 1–3, 5, 31, 49–50, 55–58, 72, 75, 106, 142, 144;
  impressionable 57, 292;
  for socialising, dating, studying or working 44

alcohol 161, 189, 197–8, 287

Anorexia Nervosa 159

answers, and the challenge of providing 33–4, 92, 227, 236, 256–8, 265, 320, 323, 352

anti-depressant medication 318

antique dealer (example of threats) 245

anxiety 21–2, 97–8, 161, 165–7, 182–3, 185–6, 188–90, 197, 211–18, 233–9;
  crippling 99;
  cycle of 224;
  and depression 1134;
  disorders 4–6;

  experiencing 215;
  extreme 13;
  heightened 162;
  levels 243–4, 285;
  managing 197;
  and obsessional disorders 6, 166;
  problems 7, 78, 166, 219, 242;
  provoking 128–9, 162, 184, 291;
  severe 21, 61, 179, 285;
  social 69;
  spiking 233, 244;
  and stress 355;
  triggering of 61;
  and unhelpful thinking 282;
  and worries 234; see also anxious thoughts

anxious thoughts 60, 112

appearance 12–21, 55–6, 59–60, 98–108, 153–6, 163–4, 173–6, 229–39, 267–74, 319–24, 319;
  and changes in 319–21;
  checking on 19;
  comparing 18;
  fluctuating of 320-1;
  and image 8;
  issues 234;
  person's 16, 157;
  problems 232;
  and setting high standards 69

apprentices 245–46

arms, and worries concerning 136, 186, 327, 338–9

assumptions 19, 113, 156, 164, 166, 172, 202–3;
  automatic 335;
  and beliefs 202–3;
  correct 133;
  and interpretations 113

226, 229, 239;
and anxiety 217;
and behaviours 212;
and re-focussing one's thinking
261;
and responses 211
unkind comments, and the effects
of 55, 123, 207, 272, 335, 339

## V

Veale, Prof. David 95–97, 344

## W

weight 12, 31–2, 45, 49, 90, 99, 115,
159
worries 62–4, 112–3, 129–30, 161,
168, 229–239, 248–53, 256–262,
326–7, 335;
and anxiety 233;
and beliefs 117;
by employees 216;
triggering of 332
worry problems 223–5, 238, 248,
326–7

## ABOUT US

Welbeck Balance publishes books dedicated to changing lives. Our mission is to deliver life-enhancing books to help improve your wellbeing so that you can live your life with greater clarity and meaning, wherever you are on life's journey. Our Trigger books are specifically devoted to opening up conversations about mental health and wellbeing.

Welbeck Balance and Trigger are part of the Welbeck Publishing Group – a globally recognized independent publisher based in London. Welbeck are renowned for our innovative ideas, production values and developing long-lasting content. Our books have been translated into over 30 languages in more than 60 countries around the world.

If you love books, then join the club and sign up to our newsletter for exclusive offers, extracts, author interviews and more information.

To find out more and to sign up, visit:
www.welbeckpublishing.com

Twitter.com/welbeckpublish
Instagram.com/welbeckpublish
Facebook.com/welbeckuk

Find out more about Trigger:
www.triggerhub.org

Twitter.com@Triggercalm
Facebook.com @Triggercalm
Instagram.com @Triggercalm

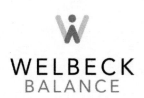

WELBECK
BALANCE